LIBRARY-LRC
TEXAS HEART INSTITUTE

ECHOCARDIOGRAPHY

Dedication

To Emily and William

ECHOCARDIOGRAPHY
A Practical Guide for Reporting

2nd edition

Helen Rimington BSc
Head of Echocardiography
Guy's and St Thomas' Hospitals, London

John B Chambers MD FESC FACC
Head of Noninvasive Cardiology
Guy's and St Thomas' Hospitals, London

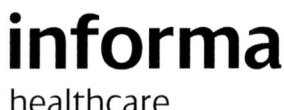

© 2007 Informa UK Ltd

First published in the United Kingdom in 1998 by The Parthenon Publishing Group Limited

Second edition published in the United Kingdom in 2007 by Informa Healthcare, Telephone House, 69-77 Paul Street, London, EC2A 4LQ. Informa Healthcare is a trading division of Informa UK Ltd. Registered Office: 37/41 Mortimer Street, London W1T 3JH. Registered in England and Wales number 1072954

Tel: +44 (0)20 7017 5000
Fax: +44 (0)20 7017 6699
Website: www.informahealthcare.com

All rights reserved. No part of this publication may be reproduced, stored in a retrieval system, or transmitted, in any form or by any means, electronic, mechanical, photocopying, recording, or otherwise, without the prior permission of the publisher or in accordance with the provisions of the Copyright, Designs and Patents Act 1988 or under the terms of any licence permitting limited copying issued by the Copyright Licensing Agency, 90 Tottenham Court Road, London W1P 0LP.

Although every effort has been made to ensure that all owners of copyright material have been acknowledged in this publication, we would be glad to acknowledge in subsequent reprints or editions any omissions brought to our attention.

A CIP record for this book is available from the British Library.
Library of Congress Cataloging-in-Publication Data

Data available on application

ISBN-10: 1 84184 634 1
ISBN-13: 978 184184 634 7

Distributed in North and South America by
Taylor & Francis
6000 Broken Sound Parkway, NW, (Suite 300)
Boca Raton, FL 33487, USA

Within Continental USA
Tel: 1 (800) 272 7737; Fax: 1 (800) 374 3401
Outside Continental USA
Tel: (561) 994 0555; Fax: (561) 361 6018
Email: orders@crcpress.com

Distributed in the rest of the world by
Thomson Publishing Services
Cheriton House
North Way
Andover, Hampshire SP10 5BE, UK
Tel: +44 (0)1264 332424
Email: tps.tandfsalesorder@thomson.com

Composition by Scribe Design Ltd, Ashford, Kent, UK
Printed and bound in India by Replika Press Pvt Ltd

CONTENTS

	Preface	vii
	Acknowledgements	viii
	List of abbreviations	ix
1	**Introduction**	1
	Minimum standard echocardiogram	1
	Organisation of a report	2
2	**Left ventricle**	5
	Systolic function	5
	Diastolic function	11
	Pericardial constriction vs restrictive cardiomyopathy	15
	Cardiac resynchronisation	17
3	**Myocardial infarction**	23
4	**Cardiomyopathies**	27
	Dilated LV	27
	Hypertrophied LV	29
	Restrictive cardiomyopathy	33
	Arrhythmogenic RV dysplasia and LV non-compaction	35
5	**Valve disease**	39
	Aortic stenosis	39
	Aortic regurgitation	42
	Mitral stenosis	46
	Mitral regurgitation	49
	Tricuspid stenosis and regurgitation	59
	Pulmonary stenosis and regurgitation	61
6	**Prosthetic valves**	65
	General	65
	Aortic position	67

Contents

	Mitral position	70
	Right-sided	72
7	**Endocarditis**	**75**
8	**Aorta**	**79**
	Aortic dilatation	79
	Before aortic valve surgery	80
	Dissection	82
	Marfan and Ehlers–Danlos syndromes	83
	Coarctation	83
9	**Atria**	**87**
10	**Right heart**	**89**
	Right ventricle	89
	Pulmonary hypertension	94
11	**Adult congenital disease**	**99**
	Simple defects	99
	Systematic study	100
	Post-procedure studies	107
12	**Pericardial effusion**	**109**
13	**Masses**	**115**
14	**General**	**119**
	Specific clinical requests	119
	Indications for urgent clinical advice	125
	Indications for further echocardiography	125

Appendices — 129
1. Normal ranges for cardiac dimensions — 129
2. Normal values for replacement heart valves — 134
3. Summary of formulae — 134
4. Body surface area nomogram — 141

Index — 143

PREFACE

This book is not a systematic textbook about echocardiography. It provides a scheme for the interpretation of a study as an aide-memoire for the experienced echocardiographer or interpreting physician and as a learning tool for the beginner.

Since the first edition, the text has been extensively revised by the inclusion of new guidelines, grading criteria, and normal data, including Doppler tissue imaging. It has also been reformatted to be more easily accessible. New chapters have been added on cardiac resynchronization and the atria. Echocardiography is increasingly used in acute medicine and the intensive therapy unit, and a chapter on checklists in clinical presentations and guides to the role of transoesophageal and stress echocardiography have been included.

This book will be relevant to all echocardiographers, including sonographers, cardiologists, intensivists, and physicians in acute, general and emergency medicine. It will also be relevant to all physicians needing to interpret reports.

HR, JBC

ACKNOWLEDGEMENTS

We are grateful to many colleagues, including Harald Becher, Cathy Head, Jamil Mayet, and Simon Ray for proof-reading sections and offering comments and suggestions. We thank Ronak Rajani for the major task of updating the Guy's and St Thomas' prosthetic valve database. We also thank Cathy Head for providing Figure 11.3b and Jane Hancock for Figure 3.1b.

ABBREVIATIONS

Ao	aorta	PDA	persistent ductus arteriosus
ARVD	arrhythmogenic right ventricular dysplasia	PFO	patent foramen ovale
ASD	atrial septal defect	PV	pulmonary vein
AV	atrioventricular	PW	posterior wall thickness
AVSD	atrioventricular septal defect	RA	right atrium
BSA	body surface area	RV	right ventricle/ventricular
ECG	electrocardiogram	RWT	regional wall thickness
EOA	effective orifice area	SVC	superior vena cava
dP/dt	rate of developing pressure	TIA	transient ischaemic attack
IVC	inferior vena cava	TOE	transoesophageal echocardiography
IVS	interventricular septal thickness	TTE	transthoracic echocardiography
LA	left atrium/atrial	V_{max}	peak velocity
LBBB	left bundle branch block	VSD	ventricular septal defect
LV	left ventricle/ventricular	VTI_1	subaortic velocity time integral
LVDD	LV diastolic dimension	VTI_2	transaortic velocity time integral
LVSD	LV systolic dimension		
PA	pulmonary artery		

1 INTRODUCTION

MINIMUM STANDARD ECHOCARDIOGRAM

- A minimum set of views and measurements is necessary for every standard echocardiogram[1,2] in order to:
  - reduce the risk of missing abnormalities
  - help minimise variability between operators and over serial studies
  - provide an instrument for quality control.
- Further views and measurements are dictated by the reason for the request or the findings at the initial study and are discussed in each chapter.
- The template below is needed before a study can be reported as normal. Note that a universal consensus does not exist for the asterisked items.

The minimum standard adult transthoracic study

Two-dimensional sections

- Parasternal long-axis.
- Parasternal long-axis views modified to show RV inflow and outflow.*
- Parasternal short-axis at the following levels:
  - aortic valve
  - mitral leaflet tips
  - papillary muscles.
- Apical views:
  - 4-chamber
  - 5-chamber
  - 2-chamber
  - long-axis.
- Subcostal views to show the RV, atrial septum, and IVC.
- Suprasternal view.*

2D or M-mode measurements

- LV dimensions from the parasternal long-axis or short-axis view:
  - septal thickness at end-diastole
  - cavity size at end-diastole
  - posterior wall thickness at end-diastole
  - cavity size at end-systole.
- Aortic root dimension.
- LA anteroposterior diameter.

Colour Doppler mapping

- For the pulmonary valve in at least one imaging plane.
- For all other valves in at least two imaging planes.
- Atrial septum in one plane.*
- Aortic arch in the suprasternal view.*

Spectral Doppler

- Pulsed Doppler at the tip of the mitral leaflets in the apical 4-chamber view. Measure the peak E and A velocities and the E deceleration time.
- Pulsed Doppler in LV outflow tract. Measure the systolic velocity integral.*
- Continuous-wave Doppler across the aortic valve in the apical 5-chamber view. Note the peak velocity.
- Continuous-wave Doppler across the tricuspid valve if tricuspid regurgitation is seen on colour Doppler. Note the peak velocity.
- Pulsed or continuous-wave Doppler in the pulmonary artery.
- Pulsed tissue Doppler at the mitral annulus.*

ORGANISATION OF A REPORT

A report should include Doppler and M-mode or 2D measurements, observations, and a short conclusion.

Measurements

- Measured intracardiac dimensions are used to:
  - diagnose pathology (e.g., dilated cardiomyopathy)
  - aid quantification of an abnormality (e.g., LV dilatation in chronic aortic regurgitation)
  - determine treatment (e.g., surgery for mitral regurgitation if systolic LV diameter >4.0 cm)
  - monitor disease progression.

- They may need to be interpreted in the light of the size and sex of the patient. Many pragmatic normal ranges are outdated, and modern data based on large populations include upper dimensions previously regarded as abnormal (see Appendix 1).

Observations
- These should be in sufficient detail to allow another echocardiographer to visualise the study.
- All parts of the heart and great vessels should be described. If it was not possible to image a region, then this should be stated. This gives the reader the confidence that a systematic study has been undertaken rather than a study focused on only a limited region of interest.
- The order should be logical, but will vary between echocardiographers and according to the type of study. The most important feature might be described first, or each anatomic region might be discussed in turn.
- Preliminary interpretations can be included where these aid understanding – for example 'rheumatic mitral valve'. The grade of stenosis or regurgitation can also be included, provided that the observations used to make the judgement are also available e.g. in the measurement section.
- No consensus exists about reporting minor abnormalities (e.g., mild mitral annulus calcification), normal variants (e.g. Chiari net), or normal findings (e.g. trivial mitral regurgitation). We suggest describing these in the text, but omitting them from the conclusion.

Conclusion
- This should integrate and summarise the measurements and observations to answer the question posed by the requestor. It should identify any abnormality (e.g. mitral regurgitation), its cause (e.g. mitral prolapse) and any secondary effects (e.g. LV dilatation and hyperactivity).
- The conclusion should be understandable by a non-echocardiographer and may need to be tailored to the likely knowledge and expectations of the requestor.
- Management advice should not routinely be given, but the referrer may not be aware of the significance of a result, and clinically important findings (page 125) should trigger a supervising clinician to contact the referrer.
- Much clinical advice requires the echocardiographic findings to be integrated with the broader clinical assessment, which is not available to the echocardiographer. However, it may be reasonable to offer implicit management advice in the report, depending on the question being asked and the qualifications of the echocardiographer, for example

- 'Echocardiographically suitable for balloon valvotomy'
- 'Echocardiographically suitable for repair'
- 'Severe mitral regurgitation with LV dilatation at thresholds suitable for surgery'.

REFERENCES

1. Sanfillippo A, Bewick D, Chan K, et al. Guidelines for the Provision of Echocardiography in Canada. Web page, 2004. http://www.csecho.ca/.
2. Chambers J, Masani N, Hancock J, Wharton G, Ionescu A. A Minimum Dataset for a Standard Adult Transthoracic Echocardiogram from the British Society of Echocardiography Education Committee. Web page, 2005. http://www.bsecho.org/.

2 LEFT VENTRICLE

SYSTOLIC FUNCTION

1. Cavity dimensions

- Measure at the base of the heart as in the minimum standard study. Normal ranges are given in Appendix 1.
- Calculate fractional shortening (FS) using M-mode or 2D LV dimensions in diastole (LVDD) and systole (LVSD):

$$FS\ (\%) = 100 \times \frac{(LVDD - LVSD)}{LVDD}$$

- Fractional shortening describes systolic function at the base of the heart. In the absence of regional wall motion abnormalities, this may represent the whole LV.

2. Regional wall motion

- Look at each arterial region in every view.
- Describe wall motion abnormalities by segment according to their systolic thickening and phase (Table 2.1 and Figure 2.1).

Table 2.1 Wall motion by phase and thickening

Score	Wall motion
1	Normal
2	Hypokinesis (<50% normal movement)
3	Akinesis (absent movement)
4	Dyskinesis (movement out of phase with the rest of the ventricle)
5	Aneurysmal

Segments should only be scored if at least half the endocardium is adequately seen. Wall motion index is calculated by dividing the total wall motion score by the number of segments scored

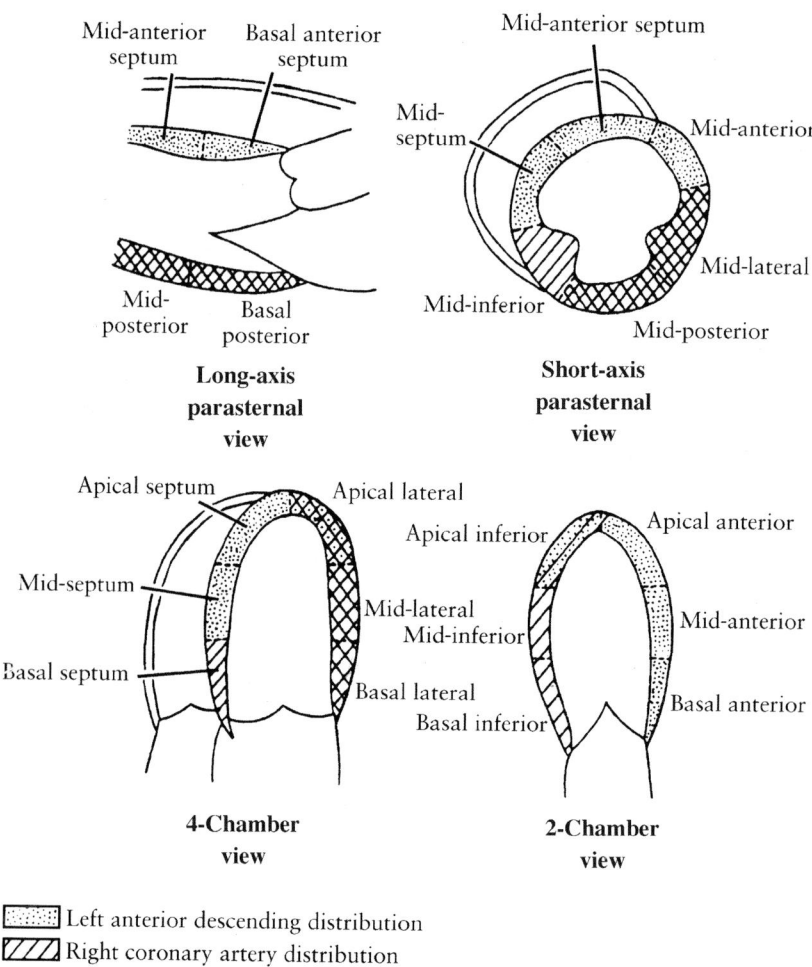

Figure 2.1 Arterial territories of the heart. The motion of the endocardium within each arterial territory should be described (Table 2.1). A 17-segment model has been proposed for myocardial contrast studies or when comparing two different imaging modalities. This has not superseded the 16-segment model for routine use (Reproduced from Segar DS et al. J Am Coll Cardiol 1992; 19: 1197–202 with permission)

3. Global function

Some measure of global function should be given. Any or all of the following may be used, depending on the preferred practice of the individual laboratory.

LV cavity volumes and ejection fraction

- With experience, the ejection fraction can be estimated by eye.[1] A value to the nearest 5% or a range (e.g., 40–50%) should be given, since the estimate can never be precise.
- Otherwise, systolic and diastolic volumes should be calculated. This can be done using the area–length method if the LV is symmetric, but the biplane modified Simpson's rule (4- and 2-chamber views) should be used if there is a wall motion abnormality.
- The ejection fraction (EF) (Table 2.2) is then given by the following expression:

$$EF\,(\%) = 100 \times \frac{\text{diastolic volume} - \text{systolic volume}}{\text{diastolic volume}}$$

- Simpson's rule should also be used if a clinical decision rests on a threshold ejection fraction (e.g., to implant a defibrillator).

Table 2.2 Grading LV function by ejection fraction[2]

Normal	Mildly abnormal	Moderately abnormal	Severely abnormal
≥55%	45–54%	30–44%	<30%

Stroke distance

- Stroke distance is the same as the subaortic velocity time integral (VTI_1) and is measured using pulsed Doppler in the LV outflow tract in the 5-chamber view.

Table 2.3 Normal ranges for subaortic velocity time integtral

	Normal[3]	Severely abnormal
Age >50	12–20	<7.0
Age <50	17–35	<11.0

- There is no firm relationship with ejection fraction, since an LV with a large diastolic volume can eject a normal volume of blood at rest even if the ejection fraction is mildly or even moderately reduced.
- Stroke volume can be calculated from stroke distance using the LV outflow tract radius ($r=$ LV outflow tract diameter/2):

  stroke volume $= \pi r^2 \times VTI_1$
- Cardiac output is given by stroke volume × heart rate.

LV dP/dt

- If mitral regurgitation can be recorded on continuous-wave Doppler, the time between 1.0 and 3.0 m/s on the upslope of the waveform allows calculation of the rate of developing pressure, dP/dt (Figure 2.2).

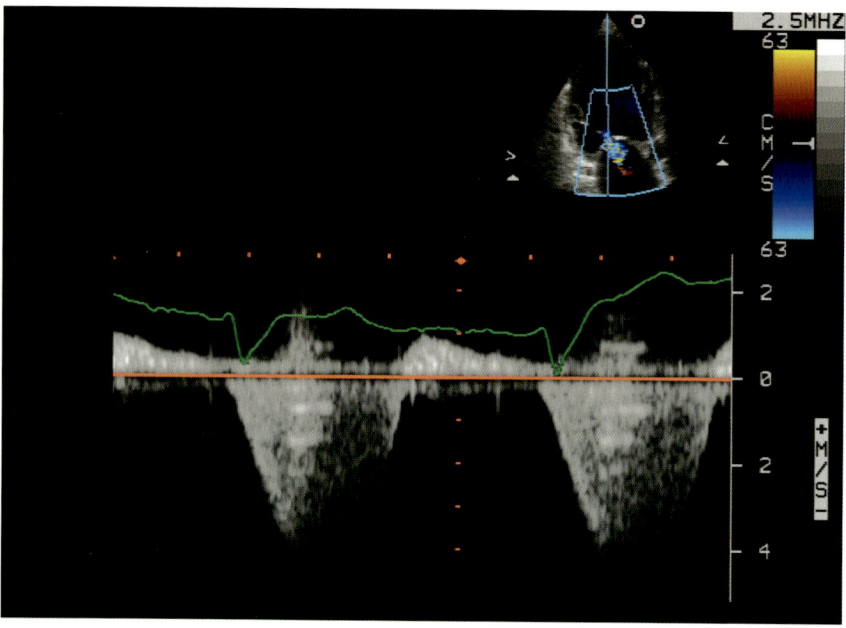

Figure 2.2 Estimating LV dP/dt. Measure the time (dt) between 1 and 3 m/s on the upstroke of the waveform which represents a pressure change of 32 mmHg [(4 ×3^2) − (4 ×1^2) using the short form of the modified Bernoulli theorem]. dP/dt is then 32/dt.

- Normal is >1200 mmHg/s which is approximately equivalent to a time between 1.0 and 3.0 m/s of ≤25 ms (Table 2.4).

Left ventricle

Table 2.4 Guide to grading LV function by mitral regurgitant signal[4]

	Normal	Mild to moderately abnormal	Severely abnormal
dP/dt (mmHg/s)	>1200	800–1200	<800
Time from 1 to 3 m/s (ms)	>25	25–40	>40

4. Long-axis function

- This should be assessed if conventional measures of systolic function are equivocal or if early signs of systolic dysfunction need to be excluded (e.g., neuromuscular disorder, family history of dilated cardiomyopathy, chronic aortic regurgitation).
- Place the Doppler tissue sample in the myocardium at the mitral annulus (Figure 2.3) and measure the peak systolic velocity (Table 2.5).
- Another method is long-axis excursion on M-mode (Figure 2.4 and Table 2.5). There is surprisingly little published information.

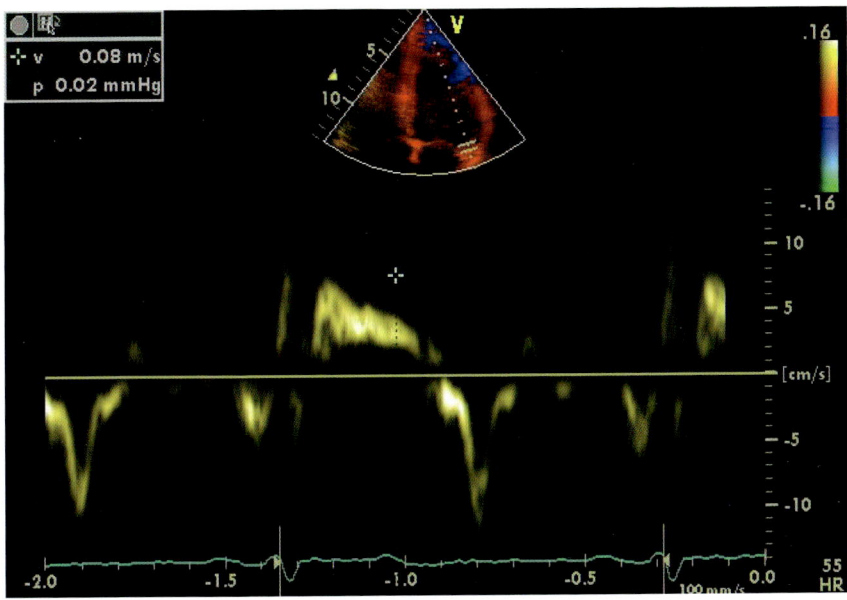

Figure 2.3 Doppler tissue imaging. The pulsed signal recorded at the lateral mitral annulus with the peak systolic velocity marked

Echocardiography: A Practical Guide for Reporting

Table 2.5 Guide to LV systolic long-axis function

	Normal	Severely abnormal
Doppler tissue peak systolic velocity (cm/s)		
Age <65	>8[5]	
Age >65	≥5[6]	
M-mode excursion (mm)		
Septal	>10	<7[7]
Lateral	>12	<7

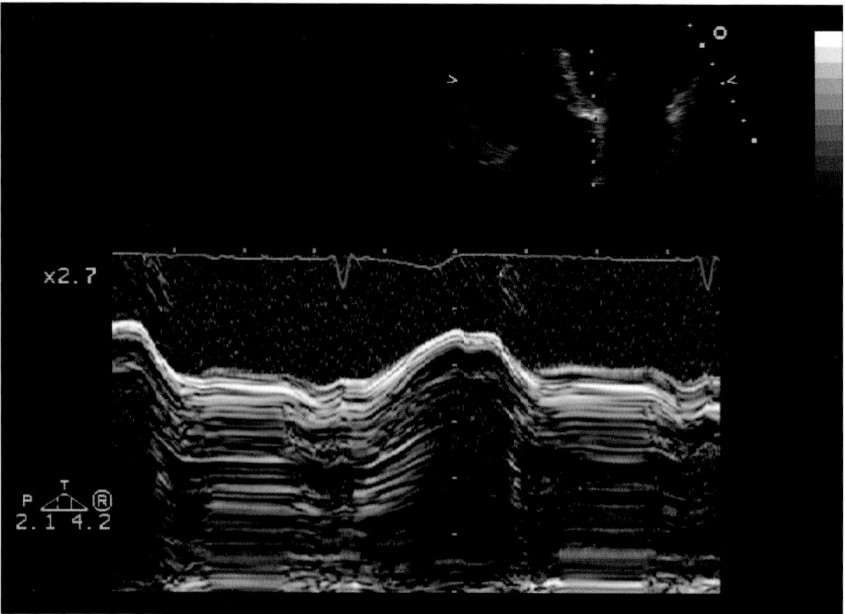

Figure 2.4 Long-axis excursion. A zoomed view of the base of the heart in a 4-chamber view is used and the M-mode cursor is placed at the lateral and septal edge (illustrated) of the mitral annulus. Long-axis excursion may be measured from the nadir (N) to the systolic peak (P) of the annulus[7]

5. Assess LV diastolic function (page 11)

- This gives information about filling pressures and prognosis. A shortened E deceleration time (<125 ms) indicates a poor prognosis, independently of systolic function.[8]

6. Other

- Complications of LV dysfunction:
  - functional mitral regurgitation (page 51)
  - thrombus (Table 3.3)
- RV function (page 89) and pulmonary pressures (page 94).

Checklist for reporting LV systolic function
1. LV cavity dimensions
2. Regional systolic function
3. Global systolic function
4. Diastolic function
5. Complications (e.g. thrombus, mitral regurgitation)
6. RV function and pulmonary pressure

DIASTOLIC FUNCTION

1. Appearance on 2D

- Is there LV hypertrophy (page 29) or a large LA (in the absence of mitral valve disease; page 87), either of which suggest that diastolic function is likely to be abnormal.

2. Pattern of mitral filling (Figure 2.5)

- Place the pulsed sample at the level of the tips of the mitral leaflets in their fully open diastolic position. Measure the peak E and A velocities and the E deceleration time. Is the pattern of filling normal, slow, or restrictive?

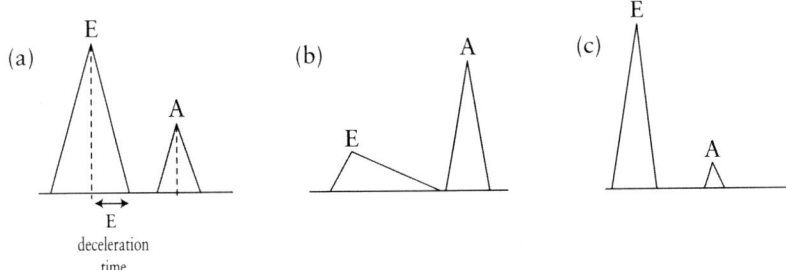

Figure 2.5 LV filling patterns: (a) normal; (b) slow filling (low peak E velocity with long deceleration time and high peak A velocity); (c) restrictive (high peak E velocity with short E deceleration time and with low or absent A wave)

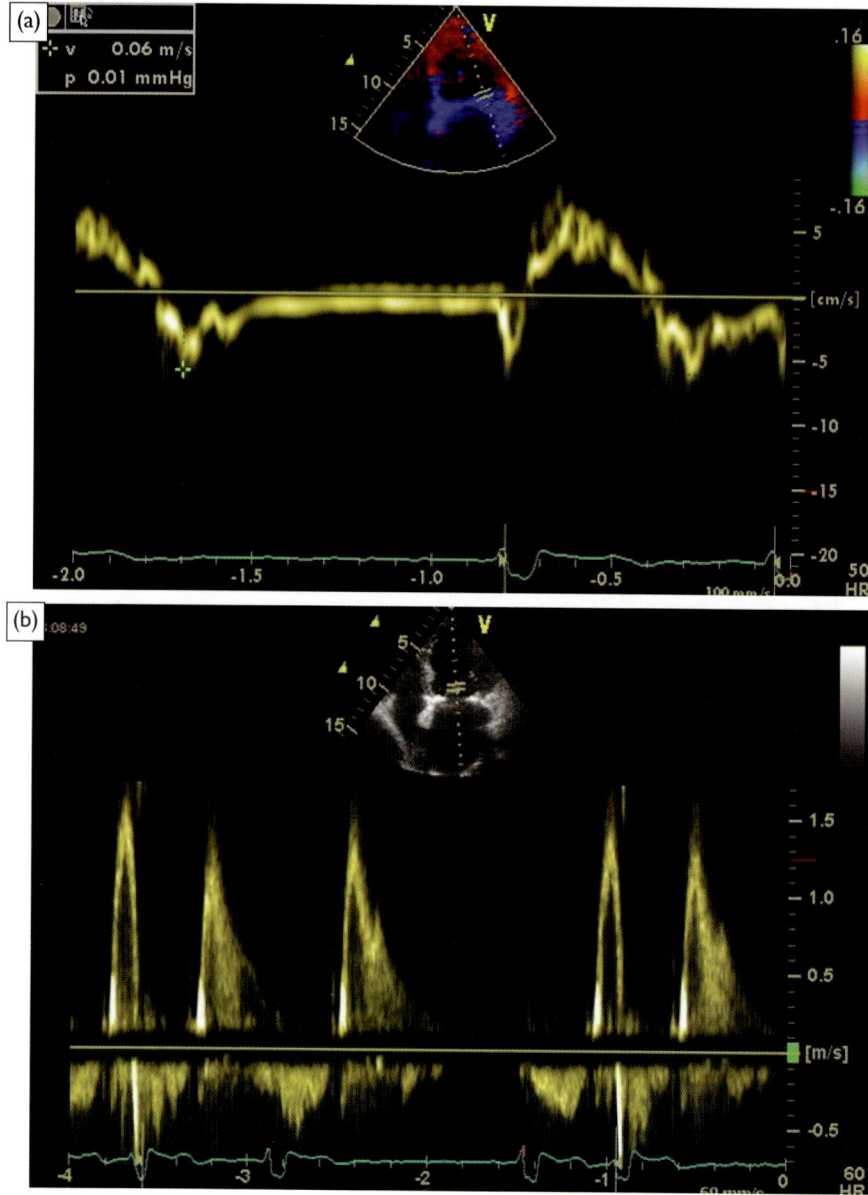

Figure 2.6 Tissue Doppler. A normal pulsed tissue Doppler recording is shown in Figure 2.3. The signals shown here were recorded from a patient admitted with pulmonary oedema, an echocardiogram showing a normal LV ejection fraction with normal coronary angiography. The tissue Doppler recording at the lateral edge of the mitral annulus (a) gave a peak E' of 6 cm/s, while the peak transmitral E velocity was 150 cm/s (b). The E/E' ratio of 25 was therefore much higher than the upper limit for normal of 10, indicating a filling pressure sufficient to cause pulmonary oedema

3. Tissue Doppler (Figure 2.6)
- Place the pulsed sample at the lateral border of the mitral annulus. Measure the peak E velocity (E' or Ea).

4. Diagnosis of diastolic dysfunction
- Categorise diastolic function using the transmitral E and A waves and the Doppler tissue E' velocity (Table 2.6).

Table 2.6 Guideline diagnosis of diastolic dysfunction

LV diastole	E/A ratio[a]	E deceleration time (ms)[a]	E/E' ratio[b]
Normal	0.7–1.5	150–250	≤10
Mild dysfunction (slow filling)	<0.7	>250	≤10
Moderate dysfunction (pseudonormal)	0.7–1.5	150–250	>10
Severe dysfunction (restrictive)	>1.5	<150	>10

[a]Precise values vary between research studies; these ranges are a composite[9-14]
[b]If tissue Doppler is recorded at the septum, a ratio of >15 is the usual cut-point[15]

- If there is a restrictive filling pattern with a normal cavity size in diastole, consider restrictive cardiomyopathy or constrictive pericarditis (see page 15).
- Restrictive filling is sometimes subdivided into reversible (normalises with a fall in preload – e.g. after a Valsalva manoeuver) and irreversible. Irreversible restrictive filling is associated with a particularly high risk of events.

5. PV flow
- Usually, the mitral filling pattern in conjunction with the tissue Doppler measures are sufficient to assess diastole but, on occasion it is necessary to measure the following (Table 2.7 and Figure 2.7):
    - the peak velocity of the pulmonary flow reversal
    - the duration of atrial flow reversal (PV duration)
    - the duration of the transmitral A wave (transmitral duration).
- The most reliable measure of diastolic dysfunction is:
    - PV duration – transmitral duration >30 ms.

14   Echocardiography: A Practical Guide for Reporting

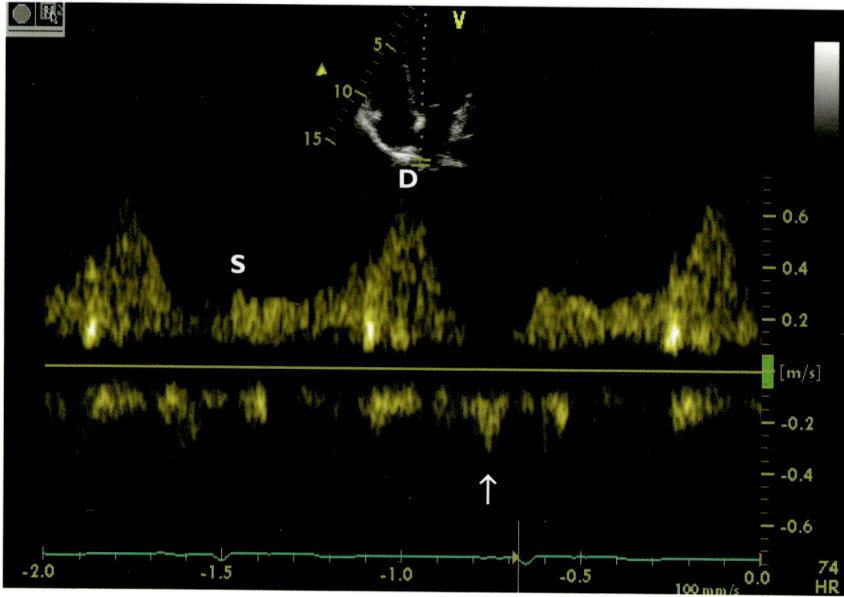

Figure 2.7 PV flow patterns. The systolic (S) and diastolic (D) peaks of forward flow are marked. Atrial reversal (arrow) has a peak velocity of 0.35 m/s

Table 2.7 Diastolic function using transmitral and PV pulsed Doppler[9–12]

	Transmitral pattern	Duration of PV A-wave reversal	PV A-wave peak velocity (m/s)
Normal	Normal	Normal	<0.35
Mild dysfunction	Slow	Normal	<0.35
Moderate dysfunction	Pseudo-normal	Prolonged (>30 ms)	>0.35
Severe dysfunction	Restrictive	Prolonged (>30 ms)	>0.35

Checklist for reporting diastolic function

1. Appearance of LV and LA
2. Transmitral filling pattern
3. Doppler tissue and, if necessary, PV flow
4. Grading of LV diastolic dysfunction

PERICARDIAL CONSTRICTION VS RESTRICTIVE CARDIOMYOPATHY (Table 2.8)

1. Features common to both

In constrictive pericarditis, the ventricles are normal and the pericardium is 'tight', while restrictive cardiomyopathy is a disease of the myocardium. However, in the early stages, the two conditions may be difficult to differentiate and may share the following features:

- a restrictive transmitral filling pattern (E/A >1.5 and an E deceleration time <150 ms)
- a normal or near-normal fractional shortening or ejection fraction
- a dilated unreactive IVC.

2. Features on the 2D study

- Biatrial enlargement occurs in both, but is usually more severe in restrictive cardiomyopathy.
- In restrictive cardiomyopathy, there may be LV hypertrophy.
- In constriction, there may be a double component to ventricular septal motion during atrial systole ('septal bounce').
- In constriction, there may be pericardial fluid or thickening (although echocardiography cannot provide an accurate assessment of pericardial thickness).

3. Left-sided respiratory variability

- Record the transmitral E wave or the peak transaortic velocities. Subtract the lowest (inspiratory) from the highest (expiratory) and express as a percentage of the highest velocity.

Table 2.8 Differentiating pericardial constriction and restrictive cardiomyopathy

Points in favour of pericardial constriction
- >25% fall in transmitral E velocity or aortic velocity on inspiration
- Tissue Doppler E' ≥ 8 cm/s
- Atria only mildly dilated
- Pulmonary vein systolic:diastolic forward velocity ratio >0.65 on inspiration and diastolic velocity falls by >40% on inspiration

Points in favour of restrictive cardiomyopathy
- <10% fall in transmitral E velocity or aortic velocity on inspiration
- Tissue Doppler E' <8 cm/s
- PA systolic pressure >50 mmHg

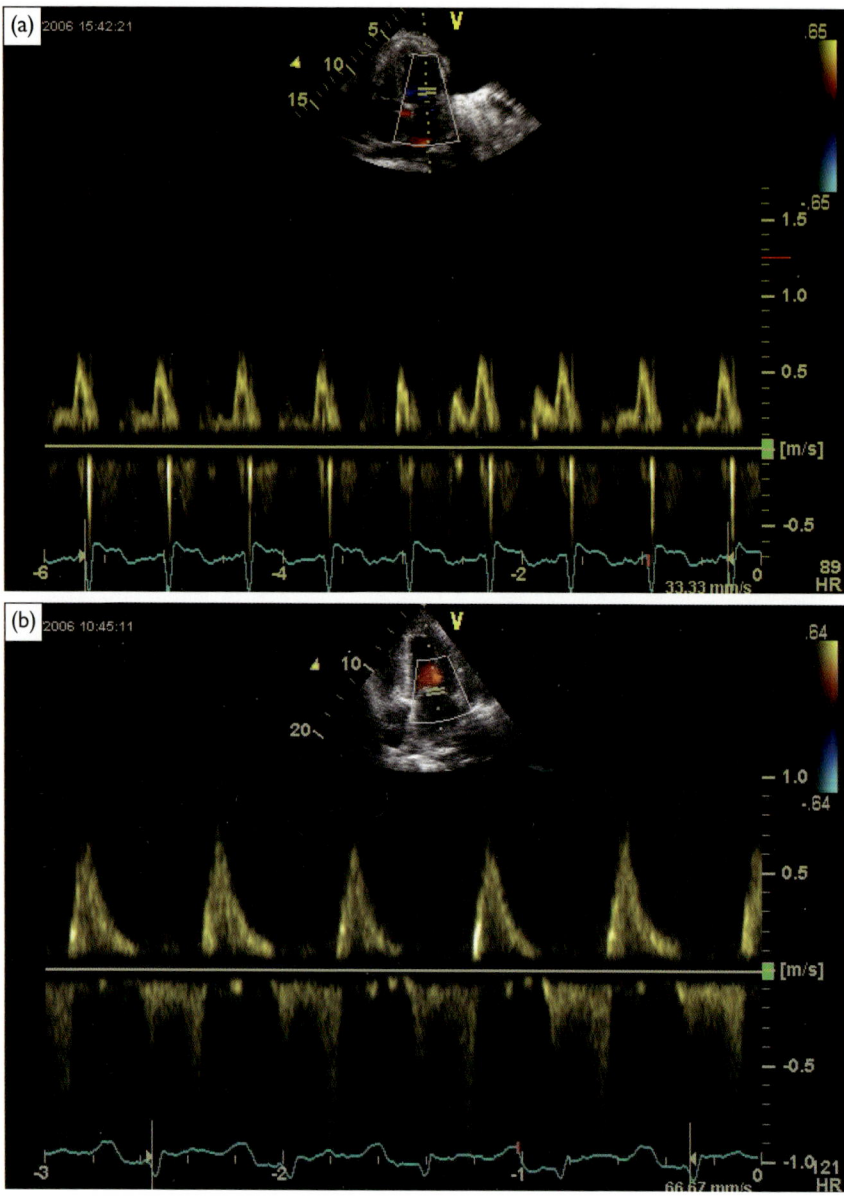

Figure 2.8 Arterial paradox. (a) This was recorded in a patient with pericardial constriction. A large left pleural effusion can be seen around the LV. The transmitral E-wave velocity was maximal (0.4 m/s) on the 7th cycle and only 0.15 m/s on the 4th cycle. The E wave was absent altogether on the 5th cycle so the fall was 100%, which is well over the threshold for abnormal of 25%. (b) This was recorded in a patient with restrictive cardiomyopathy as a result of amyloid secondary to multiple myeloma. The E wave varies little throughout the respiratory cycle

- There may be up to a 10% difference in normal subjects, usually <10% in restriction and usually >25% in constriction[16,17] (Figure 2.8).

4. Doppler tissue

- An E' at the lateral or septal annulus of ≥8 cm/s differentiates constrictive pericarditis from restrictive cardiomyopathy.[18,19]
- A low systolic velocity suggests restrictive cardiomyopathy, but may not be reliable.[19]

5. Other features

- There is an exaggerated respiratory change in pulmonary vein flow in constrictive pericarditis (systolic:diastolic forward velocity ratio >0.65 and diastolic velocity falls by >40% on inspiration).
- The pulmonary artery pressure tends to be higher in restrictive cardiomyopathy (>50 mmHg).

Checklist for reporting suspected pericardial constriction or restrictive cardiomyopathy

1. Atrial size
2. LV size and function, including septal 'bounce'
3. Pericardium, including presence of fluid
4. Transmitral and aortic flow
5. Doppler tissue at the septal or lateral mitral annulus
6. IVC size and response to inspiration

CARDIAC RESYNCHRONISATION

- There is no consensus on the relative place of echocardiography and other measures for predicting suitability for biventricular pacing, nor is there any agreement on what measures should be used. Current echocardiographic algorithms include the following:
  - LV ejection fraction
  - interventricular delay
  - intra-LV delay.

1. LV function

- Measure ejection fraction using Simpson's rule. A common threshold for cardiac resynchronisation is an ejection fraction <35%.

- Also assess regional function, since thin and scarred myocardium is unlikely to improve.

2. Interventricular delay

Individual centres use one or more of the following methods, all of which have different thresholds for predicting a response.

Delay between pulmonary and aortic flow

- Measure the time from the start of the Q wave to:
  - the onset of flow on pulsed Doppler at the pulmonary annulus
  - the onset of flow in the LV outflow tract.
- The difference between these values is the interventricular delay. A value >40 ms is currently taken as a criterion for cardiac resynchronisation therapy.

Tissue Doppler

- Measure the time from the start of the Q wave to:
  - the start of the systolic signal with the sample on the RV free wall margin of the tricuspid annulus
  - the most delayed of the posterior, lateral, and septal LV sites (see Section 3 below).
- The difference between these is the interventricular delay.
- A response is thought to be predicted by a sum asynchrony time of ≥102 ms,[20] where sum asynchrony is defined as:
(maximum – minimum LV delay) + (interventricular delay).

Septal to posterior wall delay on M-mode

- Measure the delay between the point of maximum inward motion of the septal and the posterior wall in the parasternal short or long-axis view. A delay >130 ms predicts a positive response.[21]

3. Intra-LV delay

- Measure the time from the start of the Q wave to the start of the systolic signal with the tissue Doppler sample on:
  - the lateral margin of the mitral annulus (4-chamber view)
  - the septal margin of the mitral annulus (4-chamber view)
  - the anterior margin of the mitral annulus (2-chamber view)
  - the posterior margin of the mitral annulus (2-chamber view).

Some centres also include:
- the anterior and margin of the mitral annulus (apical long-axis view)
- the posterior margin of the mitral annulus (apical long-axis view).
- The difference between the earliest and latest times is the intra-LV delay. A threshold of 65 ms suggests a benefit from cardiac resynchronisation.[21]
- Many other measures are being evaluated, including the standard deviation of regional delay to peak systolic contraction over all segments on 3D imaging.

4. Optimisation after implantation

There is no final consensus, but the following is a guide:
- Start with interventricular delay. Assess the pattern of transmitral flow, measure diastolic filling time and subaortic velocity integral on pulsed Doppler, and assess the grade of mitral regurgitation subjectively with:
  - both ventricles activated at the same time
  - the RV activated earlier than the left (e.g., 30 and 50 ms)
  - the LV activated earlier than the right (e.g., 30 and 50 ms).
- Choose the sequence with the most normal-looking transmitral filling pattern, the longest diastolic filling time, highest subaortic velocity integral, and ideally the least mitral regurgitation.
- Then optimise AV delay. Measure the diastolic filling time and the subaortic velocity integral and assess the grade of mitral regurgitation subjectively with:
  - the shortest AV delay possible
  - about 75 ms
  - about 150 ms.
- Choose the AV delay with the optimal transmitral filling pattern and velocity integral (and the least mitral regurgitation).

Checklist for reporting cardiac resynchronisation therapy study

1. LV size and function, including ejection fraction using Simpson's rule
2. Regional wall motion
3. Interventricular delay
4. Intra-left ventricular delay

REFERENCES

1. Hope MD, de la PE, Yang PC, et al. A visual approach for the accurate determination of echocardiographic left ventricular ejection fraction by medical students. J Am Soc Echocardiogr 2003; 16:824–31.
2. Lang RM, Bierig M, Devereux RB, et al. Recommendations for chamber quantification. Eur J Echocardiogr 2006; 7:79–108.
3. Rawles JM. Linear cardiac output: the concept, its measurement, and applications. In: Chambers JB, Monaghan MJ, eds. Echocardiography: An International Review. Oxford: Oxford University Press, 1993: 23–36.
4. Nishimura RA, Tajik AJ. Quantitative hemodynamics by Doppler echocardiography: a noninvasive alternative to cardiac catheterization. Prog Cardiovasc Dis 1994; 36:309–42.
5. Elnoamany MF, Abdelhameed AK. Mitral annular motion as a surrogate for left ventricular function: correlation with brain natriuretic peptide levels. Eur J Echocardiogr 2006; 7:187–98.
6. Onose Y, Oki T, Mishiro Y, et al. Influence of aging on systolic left ventricular wall motion velocities along the long and short axes in clinically normal patients determined by pulsed tissue doppler imaging. J Am Soc Echocardiogr 1999; 12:921–6.
7. Alam M, Rosenhamer G. Atrioventricular plane displacement and left ventricular function. J Am Soc Echocardiogr 1992; 5:427–33.
8. Giannuzzi P, Temporelli PL, Bosimini E, et al. Independent and incremental prognostic value of Doppler-derived mitral deceleration time of early filling in both symptomatic and asymptomatic patients with left ventricular dysfunction. J Am Coll Cardiol 1996; 28:383–90.
9. Rakowski H, Appleton C, Chan KL, et al. Canadian consensus recommendations for the measurement and reporting of diastolic dysfunction by echocardiography: from the Investigators of Consensus on Diastolic Dysfunction by Echocardiography. J Am Soc Echocardiogr 1996; 9:736–60.
10. Paulus WJ. How to diagnose diastolic heart failure. European Study Group on Diastolic Heart Failure. Eur Heart J 1998; 19:990–1003.
11. Redfield MM, Jacobsen SJ, Burnett JC Jr, et al. Burden of systolic and diastolic ventricular dysfunction in the community: appreciating the scope of the heart failure epidemic. JAMA 2003; 289:194–202.
12. Mottram PM, Marwick TH. Assessment of diastolic function: what the general cardiologist needs to know. Heart 2005; 91:681–95.
13. Nagueh SF, Middleton KJ, Kopelen HA, Zoghbi WA, Quinones MA. Doppler tissue imaging: a noninvasive technique for evaluation of left ventricular relaxation and estimation of filling pressures. J Am Coll Cardiol 1997; 30:1527–33.
14. Dokainish H, Zoghbi WA, Lakkis NM, et al. Optimal noninvasive assessment of left ventricular filling pressures: a comparison of tissue Doppler echocardiography and B-type natriuretic peptide in patients with pulmonary artery catheters. Circulation 2004; 109:2432–9.
15. Ommen SR, Nishimura RA. A clinical approach to the assessment of left ventricular diastolic function by Doppler echocardiography: update 2003. Heart 2003; 89 (Suppl 3):iii18–23.
16. Goldstein JA. Cardiac tamponade, constrictive pericarditis, and restrictive cardiomyopathy. Curr Prob Cardiol 2004; 29:503–67.
17. Maisch B, Seferovic PM, Ristic AD, et al. Guidelines on the diagnosis and management of pericardial diseases executive summary; The Task Force on the Diagnosis and Management of Pericardial Diseases of the European Society of Cardiology. Eur Heart J 2004; 25:587–610.

18. Ha JW, Ommen SR, Tajik AJ, et al. Differentiation of constrictive pericarditis from restrictive cardiomyopathy using mitral annular velocity by tissue Doppler echocardiography. Am J Cardiol 2004; 94:316–19.
19. Rajagopalan N, Garcia MJ, Rodriguez L, et al. Comparison of new Doppler echocardiographic methods to differentiate constrictive pericardial heart disease and restrictive cardiomyopathy. Am J Cardiol 2001; 87:86–94.
20. Penicka M, Bartunek J, De Bruyne B, et al. Improvement of left ventricular function after cardiac resynchronization therapy is predicted by tissue Doppler imaging echocardiography. Circulation 2004; 109:978–83.
21. Bax JJ, Abraham T, Barold SS, et al. Cardiac resynchronization therapy: Part 1 – issues before device implantation. J Am Coll Cardiol 2005; 46:2153–67, 2168–82.

3 MYOCARDIAL INFARCTION

1. Regional LV systolic function

The diagnosis is confirmed in the appropriate clinical context by a regional wall motion abnormality.

- Describe the segments affected.
- Are the segments thin? This implies a non-viable scar, while a thickness >6 mm suggests that there might be viable myocardium.
- Comment on the other regions. Compensatory hyperkinesis is a good prognostic sign. Hypokinesis of a territory other than of the acute infarct suggests multivessel disease and is a poor prognostic sign.

2. Global systolic function

- The ejection fraction and velocity integral should be described. Both give prognostic information.
- If the ejection fraction appears to be low by eye, then measure the systolic and diastolic volumes using Simpson's rule. The systolic volume refines risk, and the ejection fraction is used to guide the decision for implantable defibrillator or resynchronisation.

3. Right ventricle

- Up to 30% of all inferior infarcts are associated with RV infarction, and in 10% the RV involvement is significant.
- Estimate PA pressure.

4. Describe the mitral valve

- Mitral regurgitation is common after infarction (Table 3.1).
- A restricted posterior leaflet causing a posteriorly directed jet is common after an inferior or posterior infarction.
- 'Tenting' of both leaflets leading to a central jet occurs when there is dilatation of the mid and apical parts of the LV cavity.

5. Complications (Table 3.2)

- If there is a murmur, then check for mitral regurgitation and ventricular septal rupture. These may coexist. If there is mitral regurgitation, then consider the causes listed in Table 3.1.
- Complete or partial rupture of the papillary muscle or septal rupture should be reported directly to the responsible clinician.
- A true aneurysm complicates about 5% of all anterior infarcts and is an indicator of a poor prognosis. It must be distinguished from a false aneurysm caused by free wall rupture contained by the pericardium (Table 3.4 and Figure 3.1).

Table 3.1 Causes of mitral regurgitation after myocardial infarction

- Restricted posterior mitral leaflet (page 52)
- LV dilatation leading to 'tenting' of the mitral leaflets
- Rupture of papillary muscle or major chordae
- Mitral prolapse after minor chordal dysfunction (rare)
- Coexistent mitral valve disease

Table 3.2 Complications after myocardial infarction

- Thrombus (Table 3.3)
- Aneurysm (Figure 3.1)
- Pseudoaneurysm (Figure 3.1)
- Papillary muscle rupture
- Ventricular septal rupture

Table 3.3 Features of thrombus

- Underlying wall motion abnormality
- Cleavage plane between thrombus and LV wall
- Higher density than myocardium

Myocardial infarction

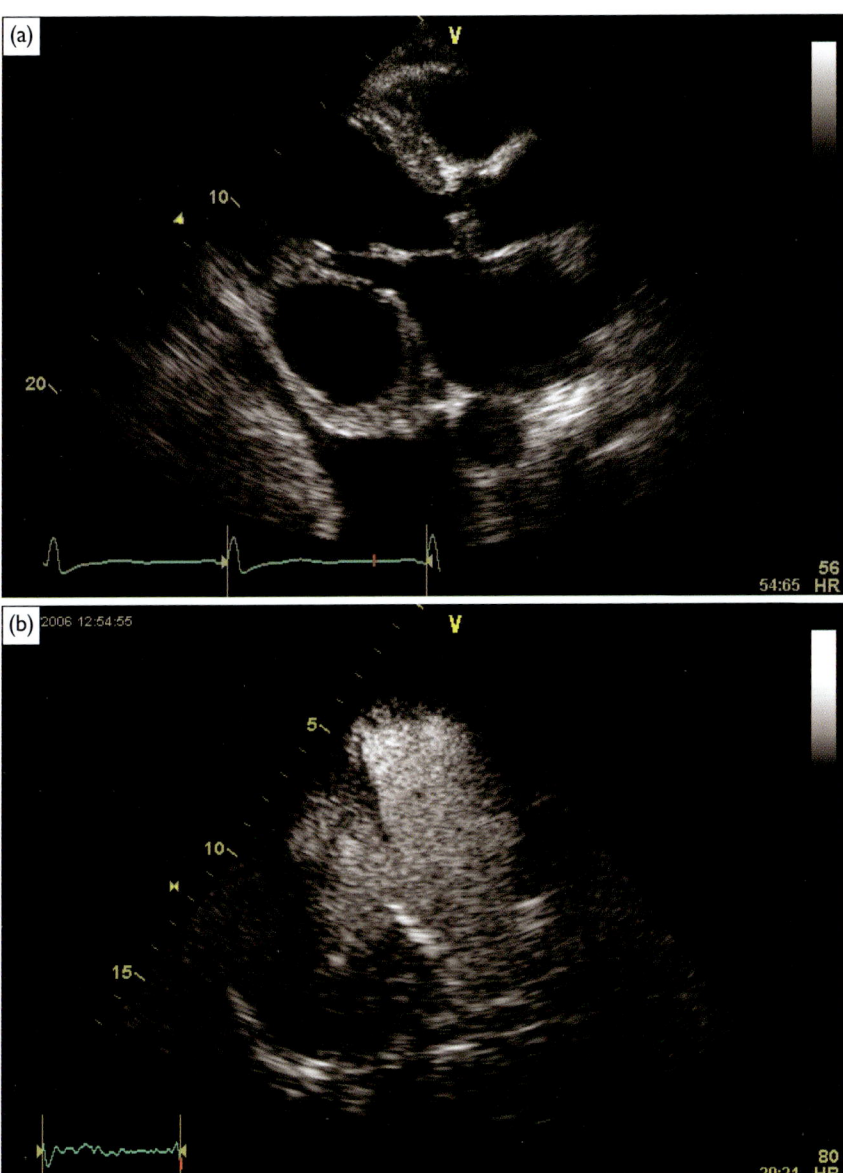

Figure 3.1
True and pseudoaneurysm. (a) A true aneurysm is caused by the infarct bulging outwards so that there is a wide neck and the myocardium is often seen in the border zone of the aneurysm. (b) A pseudoaneurysm is a rupture of the infarcted myocardial wall with blood being contained by the pericardium so that the pseudoaneurysm contains no myocardial tissue. In this example, there is a large thrombus within the cavity of the pseudoaneurysm, with a small residual space outlined by transpulmonary contrast. The inferior myocardial wall is thin and interrupted by the rupture point, which forms the usually narrow neck through which blood enters in systole and leaves in diastole

Table 3.4 Differentiation of true and pseudoaneurysm

	True aneurysm (Figure 3.1a)	Pseudoaneurysm (Figure 3.1b)
Position	More commonly apical	More commonly posterior
Neck	Wide	Narrow
Boundary	Myocardium	Pericardium
Colour flow	Swirling or absent	Into in systole, out in diastole

Checklist for reporting myocardial infarction

1. Regional wall motion
2. Global systolic function
3. RV
4. Mitral regurgitation
5. Complications

4 CARDIOMYOPATHIES

DILATED LV

Secondary myocardial impairment (e.g., as a result of hypertension) cannot be reliably differentiated from the primary cardiomyopathies on echocardiography.

1. Diagnosis using cavity dimensions and systolic function

- *Some normal ranges in use are too narrow and may result in overdiagnosis of LV dilatation, especially in large subjects.* Diastolic diameters as large as 5.9 cm may be normal (see pages 129–131).

Table 4.1 Causes of a dilated hypokinetic LV

Common
Myocardial infarction
Hypertension
Alcohol
HIV
End-stage aortic valve disease or mitral regurgitation
Ischaemic cardiomyopathy

Uncommon
Myocarditis (e.g. viral, vasculitis)
Peripartum cardiomyopathy
Neuromuscular disorders (e.g. Duchenne's muscular dystrophy)
Dilated cardiomyopathy
Sarcoid
Haemochromatosis
Cocaine
Non-compaction (Table 4.13)

- Is the LV hypokinetic (Table 4.1), normal, or hyperkinetic (Table 4.2)? Borderline hypokinesis is normal in athletic hearts (Table 4.3).

2. General appearance

- Is there a regional abnormality suggesting an ischaemic aetiology? (Figure 2.1)

Table 4.2 Causes of LV dilatation and hyperkinesis

Valve lesions
- Aortic regurgitation
- Mitral regurgitation

Shunts
- Persistent ductus
- Ventricular septal defect
- Ruptured sinus of Valsalva aneurysm

Table 4.3 Features of athletic heart[1]

- LV dilatation: diastolic diameter up to 7 cm in men and 6.6 cm in women
- Normal systolic function; occasionally borderline global hypokinesis
- Mild LV hypertrophy; septum usually ≤1.3 cm[a]
- Normal LV diastolic function
- Mild RV dilatation and hypertrophy

[a]Weightlifters and rowers may have septal thickness up to 1.6 cm

Table 4.4 Echocardiographic findings in sarcoid[2]

- Regional wall thinning especially at base of heart
- Aneurysmal dilatation
- Occasionally global LV dysfunction
- Localised mass (may involve papillary muscle, causing mitral regurgitation)
- Pericardial effusion

- Is there LV hypertrophy suggesting hypertension?
- Are both ventricles dilated suggesting a cardiomyopathy?
- Is there a valve abnormality as a possible cause of secondary myocardial impairment?
- Are there unusual features? These may include the following:
  - regional wall motion abnormality crossing arterial territories (e.g., sarcoid) (Table 4.4)
  - bright endocardial echoes (haemochromatosis)
  - apical echogenicity (consider thrombus, non-compaction)
  - abnormal myocardial density (non-specific, but consider amyloid).

3. Quantify systolic function (page 5) and assess diastolic function (page 11)

4. Are there complications?

These include the following:

- thrombus
- functional mitral regurgitation
- pulmonary hypertension.

Checklist for reporting LV dilatation

1. LV dimensions, including wall thickness
2. LV systolic and diastolic function
3. RV size and function
4. Pulmonary pressure
5. Valve function
6. Thrombus?

HYPERTROPHIED LV

1. Diagnosis and quantification of hypertrophy

- Sometimes, hypertrophy is immediately obvious – e.g. in a patient with hypertrophic cardiomyopathy (Figure 4.1). Myocardial width should then be measured at a number of points – typically in anterior, posterior, lateral and septal segments at the base and at mid-cavity level.
- More usually, the diagnosis is made after measuring wall thickness (page 129), supplemented by estimation of mass (page 139). This is

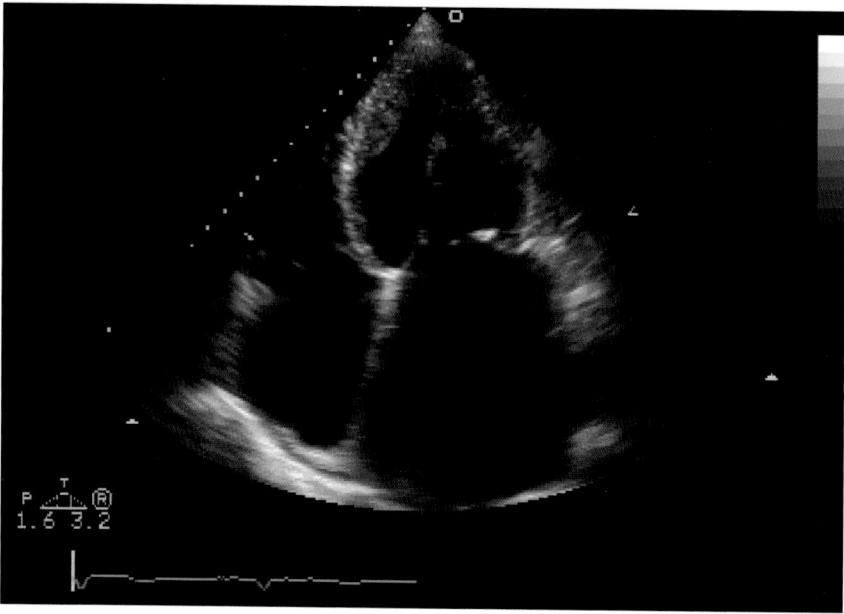

Figure 4.1 Apical hypertrophic cardiomyopathy

performed in patients with hypertension or large QRS voltages on the ECG.
- 3D and 2D methods of estimating mass are not yet widely used. An estimate can be made from linear dimensions at the base of the heart, using the following approximation:

$$0.83 \times [(LVDD + IVS + PW)^3 - LVDD^3]$$

- Mass must then be corrected for body habitus (Appendix 4), and can be used for grading hypertrophy (Table 4.5).
- Generalised hypertrophy is defined as concentric if the cavity size is small (Table 4.6).
- Concentric remodelling may develop in pressure overload even if the LV mass is normal. It is defined by a regional wall thickness (RWT) >0.45, where

$$RWT = \frac{2 \times PW}{LVDD}$$

- LV mass is not routinely estimated if there is eccentric hypertrophy, which is defined by a large cavity size and develops in volume-load (e.g. severe aortic regurgitation).

Cardiomyopathies

Table 4.5 Grading LV hypertrophy[3]

	Borderline	Moderate	Severe
Women			
LV mass (g)	163–186	187–210	≥211
LV mass/BSA (g/m^2)	96–108	109–121	≥122
IVS (cm)	1.0–1.2	1.3–1.5	≥1.6
Men			
LV mass (g)	225–258	259–292	≥292
LV mass/BSA (g/m^2)	116–131	132–148	≥149
IVS (cm)	1.1–1.3	1.4–1.6	≥1.7

Table 4.6 Causes of concentric hypertrophy[a]

Common	Uncommon
Hypertension	Hypertrophic cardiomyopathy
Aortic stenosis	Amyloid
	Storage diseases
	Friedrich's ataxia

[a]Defined as RWT >0.45.

2. Quantify systolic function and assess diastolic function

- Impaired systolic function with significant hypertrophy suggests amyloid rather than hypertrophic cardiomyopathy.
- Restrictive rather than slow or pseudonormal filling suggests amyloid.

3. Is there intracavitary or outflow tract flow acceleration?

This is assessed using continuous-wave Doppler from the apex. A peak velocity ≥2.7 m/s is a threshold for obstructive hypertrophic cardiomyopathy.[4]

4. Other signs

Look for the following:

- systolic anterior motion of the anterior leaflet of the mitral valve or of the chordae alone
- mitral regurgitation directed posteriorly away from the point of anterior motion
- abnormally long anterior mitral leaflet
- thickening of the valves
- early closure of the aortic valve.

5. Hypertrophic cardiomyopathy versus hypertension

- The diagnosis of cardiomyopathy is made using all available clinical data.
- *The echocardiography report alone should never make a new diagnosis, but can suggest hypertrophic cardiomyopathy* (Table 4.7).

Table 4.7 Hypertrophic cardiomyopathy versus hypertension: features in favour of hypertrophic cardiomyopathy

- Localised hypertrophy most frequently affecting the septum
- Hypertrophy affecting both ventricles
- Septal hypertrophy >2 cm in a non-Afro-Caribbean subject
- Abnormally long anterior mitral leaflet
- Severe systolic anterior motion of the anterior mitral leaflet
- Severe intracavitary flow acceleration
- Premature closure of the aortic valve
- Large QRS voltages and T-wave changes on the ECG

Table 4.8 Athletic heart versus mild hypertrophic cardiomyopathy: features in favour of cardiomyopathy[5]

- Asymmetric hypertrophy
- Involvement of both ventricles
- LV diastolic cavity dimension <45 mm
- Significant LA enlargement
- Diastolic dysfunction
- Female gender or family history of hypertrophic cardiomyopathy
- Abnormal ECG
- No change with detraining

Cardiomyopathies

6. Hypertrophic cardiomyopathy versus athletic heart

- Endurance athleticism usually causes mild septal thickening (≤13 mm) associated with a dilated LV cavity. Hypertrophic cardiomyopathy is not usually diagnosed unless the septal width >15 mm.
- There may be confusion if the septal width is 13–15 mm (Table 4.8).

7. Hypertrophic cardiomyopathy versus amyloid

The distinction may sometimes be difficult, but amyloid is favoured by the following:

- LV hypokinesis
- small complexes on the ECG
- valve thickening.

Checklist for reporting LV hypertrophy

1. Location of hypertrophy (check RV as well)
2. Wall thickness at representative levels
3. LV systolic and diastolic function
4. Systolic anterior motion?
5. LV outflow acceleration

RESTRICTIVE CARDIOMYOPATHY

In a patient suspected of heart failure with no obvious LV hypertrophy or dilatation and normal systolic function, consider the cardiac causes in Table 4.9.

- Look for a restrictive transmitral filling pattern and engorged IVC suggesting pericardial constriction or restrictive cardiomyopathy. These are differentiated on page 15.
- Severe bi-atrial enlargement suggests restrictive cardiomyopathy.

Table 4.9 Cardiac causes of suspected heart failure with an apparently normal LV

- Restrictive cardiomyopathy
- Constrictive pericarditis
- RV dysfunction (page 89)
- Pulmonary hypertension (page 94)

- Look for features suggesting the cause of restrictive cardiomyopathy, of which amyloid is the most common (Table 4.10).

Table 4.10 Restrictive cardiomyopathies

Cause	Comment
Secondary – infiltrative	
Amyloid	See Table 4.11
Sarcoid	See Table 4.4
Post-irradiation	Valve thickening. Combined constriction
Secondary–storage disease	
Haemochromatosis	Endocardial echogenicity
Glycogen storage	
Fabry's disease	
Primary	
Endomyocardial fibrosis	See Table 4.12
Loeffler's endocarditis	See Table 4.12
Idiopathic	

Table 4.11 Features of amyloid

- Hypertrophy affecting both ventricles
- LV hypokinesis
- Heterogeneous myocardial texture
- Restrictive filling
- Generalised valve thickening

Table 4.12 Features of endomyocardial fibrosis and Loeffler's endocarditis

- Echogenicity at RV or LV apex
- Subvalvar LV or RV thickening
- Tricuspid or mitral regurgitation
- LV or RV thrombus

Cardiomyopathies 35

> **Checklist for reporting restrictive cardiomyopathy**
>
> 1. LV size and systolic function
> 2. LV diastolic function
> 3. Respiratory variability of transmitral and subaortic flow
> 4. Valve appearance and function
> 5. IVC size and response to respiration

ARRHYTHMOGENIC RV DYSPLASIA AND LV NON-COMPACTION

1. If the LV apex is abnormally thickened

Consider the following:

- thrombus
- apical hypertrophic cardiomyopathy (Figure 4.1)
- endomyocardial fibrosis (Table 4.12)
- non-compaction (Table 4.13 and Figure 4.2).

Table 4.13 Features of isolated left ventricular non-compaction[6,7]

- Numerous, large trabeculae (usually at apex, mid-inferior, or free wall) with deep intratrabecular recesses (confirmed on colour mapping)
- Ratio of non-compacted (trabeculae) to compacted (underlying muscle) >2 on a systolic parasternal short-axis view
- Absence of congenital causes of pressure load (e.g. LV outflow obstruction)

Associated features
- Hypokinesis of affected segments
- Dilatation and hypokinesis of unaffected segments usually at the base of the LV
- Abnormal ECG (LBBB, poor R-wave progression, pathologic Q waves)

2. Isolated RV dilatation?

Consider the following:

- RV infarct
- dilated cardiomyopathy confined to the RV
- pulmonary hypertension
- ARVD (Table 4.14 and Figure 10.1).

Echocardiography: A Practical Guide for Reporting

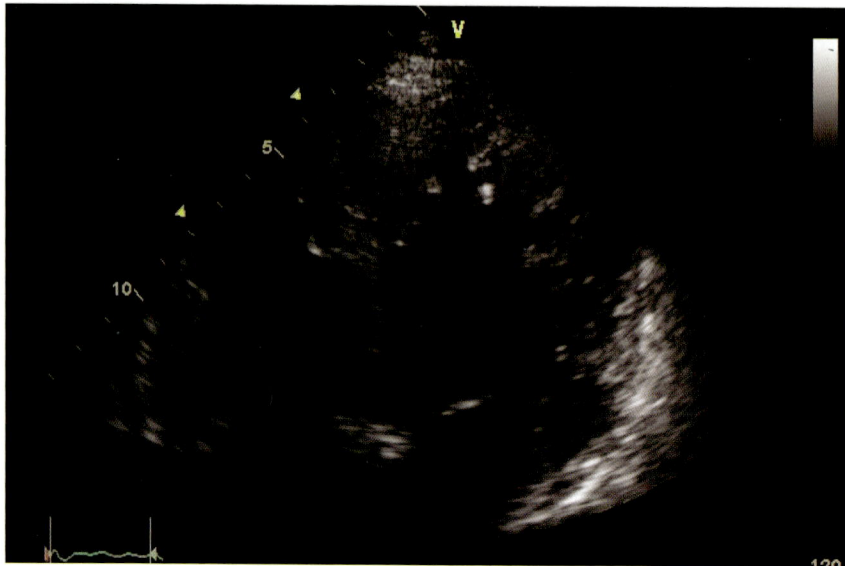

Figure 4.2 Non-compaction: This 4-chamber view was recorded in a 28-year-old woman reporting breathlessness

Table 4.14 Echocardiographic features of ARVD[8]

- General RV dilatation and hypokinesis (Figure 10.1)
- Localised RV aneurysms
- Segmental RV dilatation
- Regional RV hypokinesis (most commonly inflow, outflow, and apex)
- In advanced cases, LV involvement usually mild

Checklist for reporting arrhythmogenic RV dysplasia and LV non-compaction

Arrhythmogenic RV dysplasia
1. RV dimensions and function (page 89 and Appendix 1)
2. Exclude pulmonary hypertension and other causes of RV dilatation (page 90)

Non-compaction
1. Site of trabeculation
2. Length of trabeculation compared with myocardium
3. LV systolic and diastolic function
4. Exclude other congenital anomalies
5. Complications (e.g. thrombus, mitral regurgitation).

REFERENCES

1. Fagard R. Athlete's heart. Heart 2003; 89:1455–61.
2. Doughan AR, Williams BR. Cardiac sarcoidosis. Heart 2006; 92:282–8.
3. Lang RM, Bierig M, Devereux RB, et al. Recommendations for chamber quantification. Eur J Echocardiogry 2006; 7:79–108.
4. Maron BJ, McKenna WJ, Danielson GK, et al. American College of Cardiology/European Society of Cardiology clinical expert consensus document on hypertrophic cardiomyopathy. A report of the American College of Cardiology Foundation Task Force on Clinical Expert Consensus Documents and the European Society of Cardiology Committee for Practice Guidelines. J Am Coll Cardiol 2003 42:1687–713.
5. Maron BJ. Distinguishing hypertrophic cardiomyopathy from athlete's heart: a clinical problem of increasing magnitude and significance. Heart 2005; 91:1380–2.
6. Jenni R, Oechslin E, Schneider J, Attenhofer JC, Kaufmann PA. Echocardiographic and pathoanatomical characteristics of isolated left ventricular non-compaction: a step towards classification as a distinct cardiomyopathy. Heart 2001; 86:666–71.
7. Oechslin E, Jenni R. Isolated left ventricular non-compaction: increasing recognition of this distinct, yet 'unclassified' cardiomyopathy. Eur J Echocardiogr 2002; 3:250–1.
8. Bleeker GB, Steendijk P, Holman ER, et al. Acquired right ventricular dysfunction. Heart 2006; 92 (Suppl 1):i14–18.

5 VALVE DISEASE

AORTIC STENOSIS

1. Appearance of the valve
- Look at the number of cusps, pattern of thickening and mobility. These may give a clue to the aetiology (Table 5.1).

Table 5.1 Clues to the aetiology in aortic stenosis

	Systolic bowing	Closure line	Associated features
Calcific degenerative	No	Central	Calcification of mitral annulus or aorta
Bicuspid	Yes	Eccentric	Ascending aortic dilatation, coarctation
Rheumatic	Yes	Central	Mitral involvement

2. Assess the LV
- *If the LV is hypokinetic, the transaortic pressure difference may underestimate the grade of the stenosis, and the continuity equation should be employed.*
- Consider dobutamine stress (see Section 6) if there is apparently moderate aortic stenosis with an impaired LV.

3. Doppler measurements
- Record the continuous waveform using the stand-alone probe from the apex and at least one other approach (usually suprasternal or right intercostal) unless the aortic valve disease is obviously mild as shown by:
  - mobile cusps
  - low transaortic velocities (V_{max} <3.0 m/s)
  - a normal LV ejection fraction.

- If the continuous-wave peak velocity V_{max} <3.5 m/s, use the long form of the Bernoulli equation (Appendix 3.1) for estimating the pressure difference.
- Use the continuity equation (Appendix 3.2) to calculate the effective orifice area (EOA) – ideally in all cases, but especially if:
  - continuous-wave Doppler suggests moderate aortic stenosis (V_{max} = 3–4 m/s), since the EOA may change the grade of stenosis
  - the LV is hypokinetic.

4. Assess severity

- If the aortic valve is thickened with V_{max} <2.5 m/s (with normal LV systolic function), report 'aortic valve thickening with no stenosis'. If V_{max} ≥2.5, grade as in Table 5.2.
- Base the assessment on all available observations

Table 5.2 Severity in aortic stenosis

	Mild	Moderate	Severe
V_{max} (m/s)	2.5–3.0	3.0–4.0	>4.0
Peak gradient (mmHg)	<40	40–65	>65
Mean gradient (mmHg)	<25	25–40	>40
EOA (continuity equation) (cm^2)[1]	>1.2	0.8–1.2	<0.8

- Moderate stenosis must be interpreted carefully:
  - An area 1.0–1.5 cm^2 is moderate and <1.0 cm^2 severe by American criteria.[2]
  - The significance of the EOA depends partly on body size. An EOA <0.6 cm^2/m^2 is a threshold for severe stenosis, allowing for body surface area
  - Ultimately, management depends on clinical factors more than on the exact EOA.

5. General

- Grade aortic regurgitation (page 46).
- Assess the other valves. Functional mitral regurgitation may develop in severe aortic stenosis as the LV starts to dilate. Mitral surgery is likely to be necessary if the mitral valve is anatomically abnormal (e.g., prolapsing) or the regurgitation is more than moderate.

- Assess the aorta (page 79). Aortic root dilatation and coarctation are associated with a bicuspid aortic valve.
- Estimate the PA pressure. Pulmonary hypertension is an indicator of a poor prognosis in severe aortic stenosis.
- If there is a discrepancy in the pressure difference and the appearance of the valve, check for a subaortic membrane.

6. Low-flow aortic stenosis

- This is defined as:
  - EOA <1 cm^2, and
  - mean gradient <30 mmHg, and
  - LV ejection fraction <40%.
- The EOA may be lower than expected for the grade of stenosis as a result of the LV being unable to generate enough energy to open the valve.
- These patients need dobutamine stress echocardiography. This requires medical supervision because of the risk of cardiac arrhythmia, although this risk is not great at low infusion rates.
  - Give 5 then 10 µg/kg/min dobutamine (occasionally 20 µg/kg/min, especially if there has been prior beta-blockade).
  - Stop the infusion if the subaortic velocity time integral rises >20% or the heart rate increases.
  - Judge the severity of aortic stenosis and whether there is LV contractile reserve (Table 5.3).

Table 5.3 Stress echocardiography in low-flow aortic stenosis[3-5]

Is there severe aortic stenosis?
Mean gradient >30 mmHg and EOA <1.2 cm^2 at any time during the infusion

Is there LV contractile reserve?
Subaortic velocity time integral (or ejection fraction) rises by >20%

Checklist for reporting aortic stenosis

1. Appearance and movement of the aortic valve
2. Grade of stenosis
3. Grade of associated regurgitation
4. Size of aorta and check for coarctation
5. LV dimensions and systolic function
6. Other valves
7. Right ventricular function, including PA pressure

AORTIC REGURGITATION

1. Appearance of the valve and aortic root
- This may allow determination of the aetiology (Table 5.4).
- Measure the aorta at every standard level (see page 81).

2. Colour flow mapping
- Measure the jet height 0.5–1.0 cm below the cusps (on 2D or colour M-mode) (Figure 5.1) and express as a percentage of the diameter of the LV outflow tract.
- If the jet is eccentric, the width must be taken perpendicular to its axis. If it is so eccentric that it impinges on the septum or anterior mitral leaflet, the method is unreliable.
- The width of the narrowest portion of the jet (the vena contracta) is a reasonable alternative measurement (see Table 5.5 and Figure 5.1).

3. Continuous-wave signal
- Record either from the apex or, if the jet is directed posteriorly, from the parasternal position.
- Measure the pressure half-time and note the density of the signal compared with the density of forward flow.

4. The left ventricle
- Is the LV hyperdynamic (suggesting severe aortic regurgitation)? Chronic severe regurgitation usually causes LV diastolic dilatation. In acute regurgitation, the LV diastolic volume may be normal.
- What is the fractional shortening? If it is <25%, this suggests a relatively poor outcome.
- An LV systolic diameter >5 cm or 2.5 cm/m^2 is an indication for surgery, even in the absence of symptoms.[6,7]

5. Flow reversal at the arch
- From the suprasternal notch, describe:
  - whether flow reversal is holodiastolic, fills approximately half of diastole or is only seen at the start of diastole using colour M-mode (Figure 5.2) or pulsed Doppler (Figure 5.3)
  - how far down the aorta can flow reversal be detected on colour mapping

Table 5.4 Aetiology of aortic regurgitation

Ascending aortic dilatation	• Arteriosclerosis, Marfan syndrome, dissection
Valve	• Bicuspid Rheumatic Calcific degenerative
	• Endocarditis Prolapse Trauma
	• Rare e.g. systemic lupus erythematosus, Behçet syndrome, ankylosing spondylitis

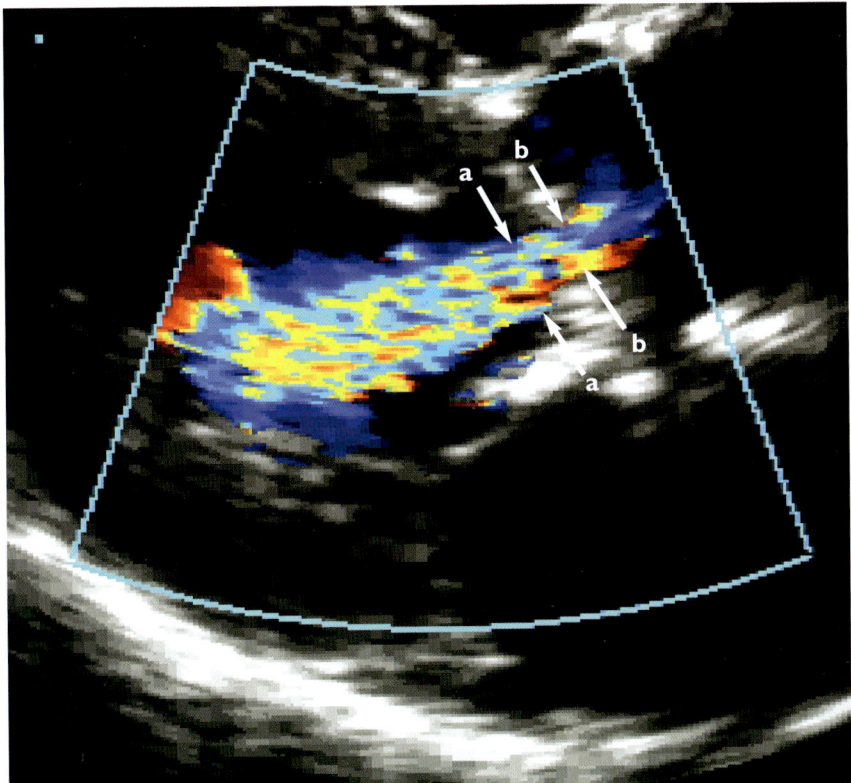

Figure 5.1 Regurgitant jet. Parasternal long-axis view. The position for measuring the height of the colour flow map as a percentage of the outflow tract height is at (a). The vena contracta or neck is at (b)

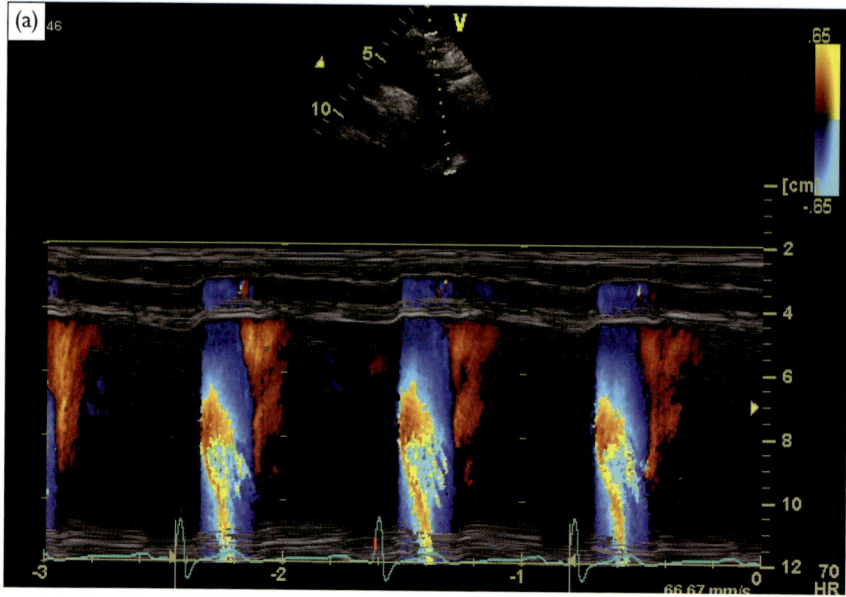

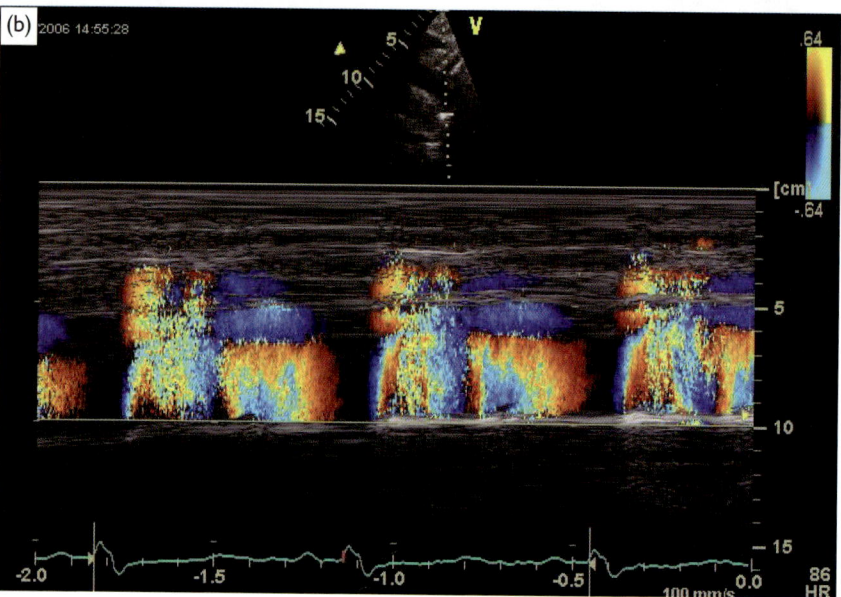

Figure 5.2 Flow reversal on colour mapping in the upper descending thoracic aorta. (a) Using suprasternal colour M-mode in a patient with mild regurgitation there is localised and short-lived flow reversal. (b) In severe regurgitation, flow reversal is holodiastolic across the whole aortic lumen and is seen well down the descending thoracic aorta

Valve disease 45

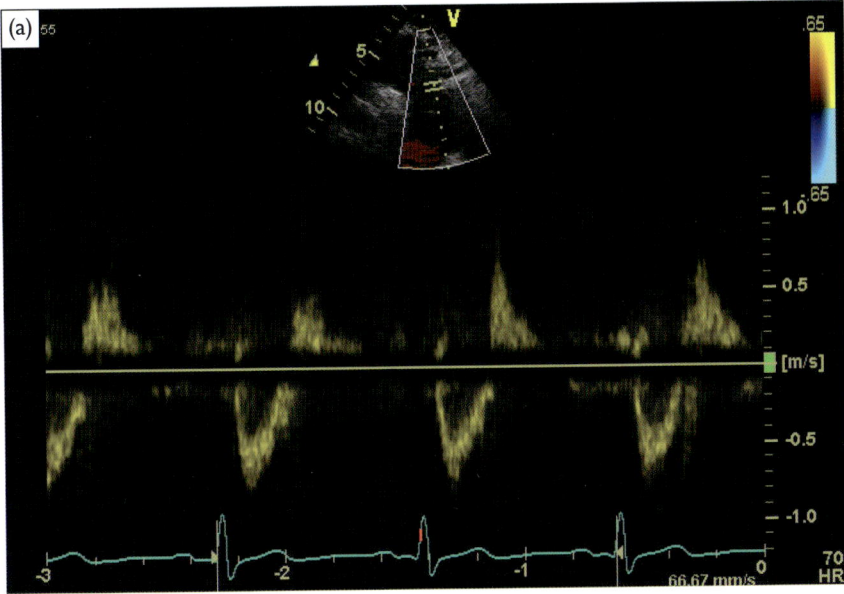

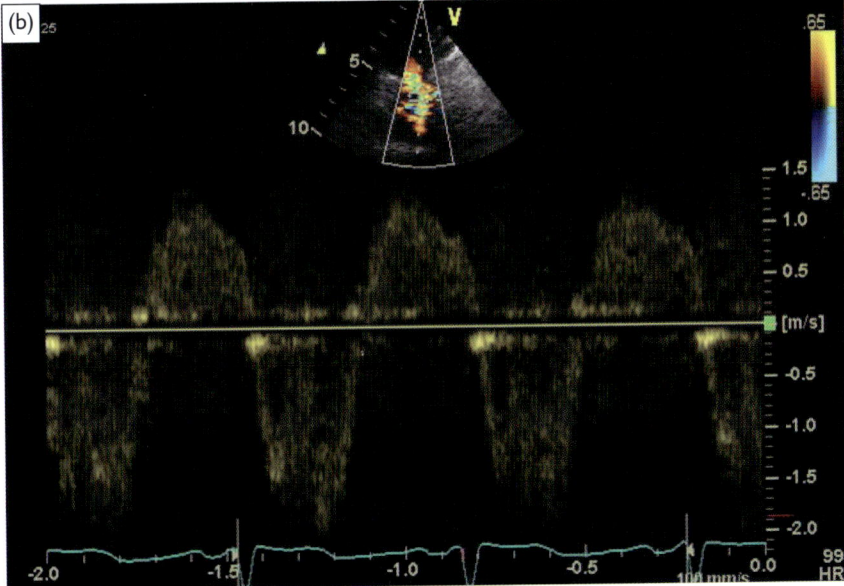

Figure 5.3 Flow reversal on pulsed Doppler in the distal arch. Using a suprasternal position. Mild regurgitation can be seen to cause short-lived low-velocity reversal (a), while in severe regurgitation the reversal is holodiastolic with a relatively high velocity at the end of diastole (e.g. ≥0.2 m/s) (b)[12]

Table 5.5 Criteria of severity in aortic regurgitation[2,8–12]

	Mild	Moderate	Severe
Colour/LV outflow tract height (%)	<25	25–64	≥65
Vena contracta width (mm)	<3	3–6	>6
Flow reversal in descending aorta	None	Not holodiastolic	Holodiastolic
Continuous-wave signal intensity	Faint or incomplete waveform	Intermediate	Dense as forward flow

6. Grade the severity of regurgitation

- Make an assessment based on all modalities. The height of the colour jet in the LV outflow tract and flow reversal beyond the arch are the most reliable modalities (Table 5.5).
- Also take into account LV size and activity.
- *The pressure half-time depends on LV diastolic function and systemic vascular resistance as well as the severity of aortic regurgitation. A cut-off of 300 ms is sensitive for severe regurgitation, but will include some patients with moderate regurgitation.*

6. Assess the other valves

- Functional mitral regurgitation may occur secondary to LV dilatation.

Checklist for reporting aortic regurgitation

1. Appearance of aortic valve
2. Grade of regurgitation
3. Aortic dimensions
4. LV dimensions and systolic function
5. Mitral valve function

MITRAL STENOSIS

1. Appearance of the valve

- Distribution and degree of thickening of both leaflets.

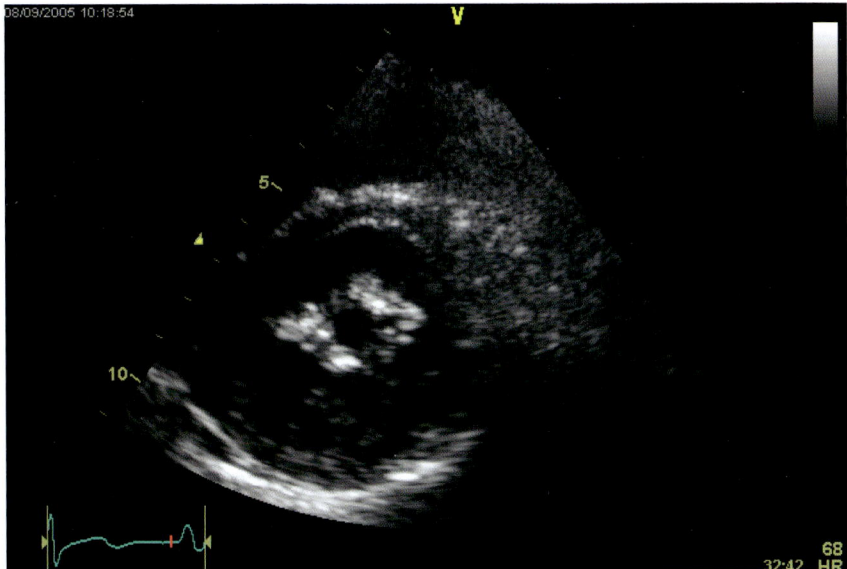

Figure 5.4 Planimetry of the mitral orifice. The orifice is imaged in a parasternal short-axis view. Care must be taken to section the tips of the mitral leaflets perpendicularly. A common mistake is to section towards the base of the leaflets or across thickened chordae

- Is there heavy echogenicity in the line of fusion of each commissure?
- Mobility of the leaflets.
- Degree of chordal involvement.

2. Planimeter the orifice area (Figure 5.4)

- Make sure that the section is not oblique.
- Use colour Doppler as a guide to the extent of the orifice if this is not obvious on imaging.
- Take care not to include the chordae, which if thickened can mimic the orifice.
- If there is significant reverberation artefact, the measurement may be inaccurate and should not be made.

3. Continuous wave signal

- Measure the pressure half-time and mean gradient, averaging 3–5 cycles if there is atrial fibrillation.
- The Hatle formula (orifice area = 220/pressure half-time) is an approximate guide to severity in moderate or severe stenosis.

4. Estimate PA pressure (page 94)

- This has a loose relationship with the severity of mitral stenosis, but pulmonary hypertension is a criterion for surgery or balloon valvotomy:[13]
  - PA systolic pressure >50 mmHg at rest.
  - PA systolic pressure >60 mmHg after exercise.

5. Assess mitral regurgitation (page 52)

- Anything more than mild means that the valve is not suitable for valvotomy.

6. Assess severity of mitral stenosis (Table 5.6)

- The planimetered orifice area is the only flow-independent measure:
  - *The pressure half-time will be shortened disproportionate to the orifice area if there is severe mitral or aortic regurgitation.*
  - *The mean gradient will increase with mitral regurgitation.*

Table 5.6 Criteria of severity in mitral stenosis

	Mild	Moderate	Severe
Orifice area by planimetry (cm^2)	>1.5	1.0–1.5	<1.0
Pressure half-time (ms)	<150	150–220	>220
Mean gradient (mmHg)	<5	5–10	>10[a]
PA pressure (mmHg)[b]	<30	30–50	>50

[a] >15 mmHg after exercise
[b] The relationship with valvar stenosis is not tight

7. Assess the other valves

- *Tricuspid rheumatic involvement is common, but easily missed.*
- Significant aortic valve disease suggests that double valve replacement rather than balloon mitral valvotomy is indicated.

8. Assess RV function

- A dilated RV is an indication for surgery or balloon valvotomy, even if there is relatively minor breathlessness.

9. Is there intra-atrial thrombus?

- TTE is insensitive for detecting thrombus. A TOE should always be performed before balloon valvotomy.
- A dilated LA >5.5 cm is used as a criterion for warfarin in the presence of sinus rhythm despite severe mitral stenosis.[13]

10. Is the valve suitable for balloon valvotomy?

- The most reliable characteristics of the valve for predicting success without developing severe mitral regurgitation are given in Table 5.7.[14,15] Some centres use the Wilkins system of scoring 1–4 for valve mobility, thickening, calcification, and subvalvar involvement (Table 5.8). A total score ≤8 suggests a successful result.[16]

Table 5.7 Markers of successful balloon valvotomy

- Good mobility of the anterior leaflet
- Minor chordal involvement (contrast Figure 5.5)
- No more than mild mitral regurgitation
- No commissural calcification (contrast Figure 5.5)
- No left atrial thrombus (on TOE)

Checklist for reporting mitral stenosis
1. Appearance of valve
2. Severity of stenosis and regurgitation
3. Right-sided pressures and RV function
4. Other valves
5. Is the valve suitable for balloon valvotomy?

MITRAL REGURGITATION

1. Appearance and movement of the valve (Table 5.9)

- Is there thickening of the leaflet? Thickening primarily involves the tips in rheumatic disease, but is more generalised in antiphospholipid syndrome or late after radiation. A floppy valve has generalised thickening that is often more obvious in one part of the cycle than another and is often associated with lax chordae

- Is there evidence of prolapse (Table 5.10) and which parts of the leaflets are involved (Figure 5.6)? Is the prolapse minor, moderate (like a bucket handle), or severe (associated with a flail tip and sometimes a visible ruptured chord)?
- Does the valve open normally during diastole, or is there bowing of the leaflets suggesting rheumatic disease?
- Is there restriction of motion of the leaflets during systole? (Table 5.11). If so, then look for LV inferoposterior infarction or global LV systolic dysfunction.
- Is there a discrete echogenic mass (e.g. vegetation or ruptured chord)?

Table 5.8 Wilkins score

Morphology	Score
Mobility	
Highly mobile, only tips restricted	1
Normal mobility of base and mid-leaflet	2
Valve moves forward in diastole mainly from the base	3
No or minimal movement	4
Leaflet thickening	
Near-normal	1
Thickening mainly at tips	2
Thickening (5–8 mm) over the whole leaflet	3
Severe thickening (>8 mm) of whole leaflet	4
Subvalvar thickening	
Minimal just below leaflets	1
Over one-third the chordae	2
Extending to the distal third of the chordae	3
Extensive thickening and shortening of the whole chord	4
Calcification	
A single area of echogenicity	1
Scattered areas at leaflet margin	2
Echogenicity extending to midportion of leaflets	3
Extensive echogenicity over whole leaflet	4

Valve disease

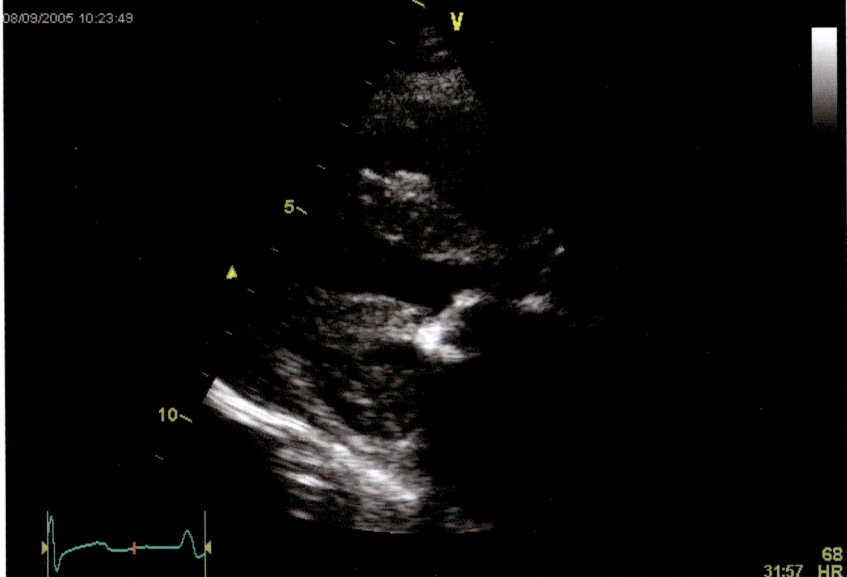

Figure 5.5 Commissural calcification and chordal involvement. This is a parasternal long-axis view angled towards the right to show the medial commissure, which contains dense calcification. The chordae are heavily matted, and it is difficult to see the junction with the papillary muscles or the mitral leaflets

Table 5.9 Aetiology of mitral regurgitation

Functional
- Global LV dilatation causing restriction of both mitral leaflets
- Regional inferoposterior wall motion abnormality causing restriction of the posterior leaflet

Ischaemic
- Acute papillary muscle or occasionally chordal rupture

Organic (abnormal mitral valve)
- Floppy mitral valve
- Endocarditis
- Rheumatic
- Other (e.g. systemic lupus erythematosus, congenital)

Table 5.10 Signs of prolapse

Prolapse is defined by either:
- movement of part of either leaflet behind the plane of the annulus in any view other than the 4-chamber view (Figure 5.7a), or
- displacement of the point of coaption behind the plane of the annulus in the 4-chamber view

Prolapse is associated with
- annular dilatation, leaflet thickening or elongation
- regurgitation, usually directed away from the prolapsing leaflet (Figure 5.7b)

Table 5.11 Restricted leaflet motion

Both leaflets
- Tenting (point of apposition above the plane of the annulus in the 4-chamber view)
- Centrally directed jet of regurgitation (Figure 5.8)
- Dilated LV, causing abnormal papillary muscle function

Restriction of posterior leaflet motion
- Tip of leaflet held in LV during systole (best seen in a long-axis view) (Figure 5.9a)
- Jet directed posteriorly (Figure 5.9b)
- Inferior or posterior infarct

Table 5.12 Grading mitral regurgitation

	Mild	Moderate	Severe
Neck width (mm)	<3	3–6.9	≥7
Flow convergence zone	Absent	Moderate	Large
EROA (mm^2)	<20	20–40	>40
Regurgitant volume (ml)	<30	30–60	>60

EROA, effective regurgitant orifice area using the PISA method

Valve disease   53

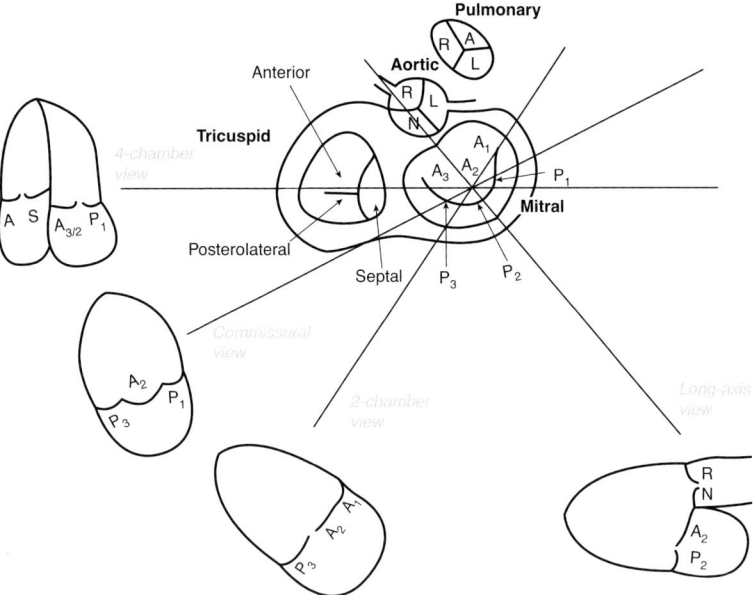

Figure 5.6 Mitral valve segments on TTE. This scheme includes a view through the commissures adapted from TOE. This can often be obtained transthoracically by slight angulation and rotation from the apical 2-chamber view

2. Colour flow mapping

Describe:
- The origin of the jet (e.g., medial, central or lateral part of the orifice).
- The direction of the jet:
  - away from a prolapsing leaflet (Figure 5.7b)
  - behind a restricted leaflet (Figure 5.9b)
  - centrally if there is symmetric 'tenting' of the leaflets (Figure 5.8) or usually in rheumatic disease.
- The size of the flow recruitment area in the LV by eye or using the PISA method if this is local policy (Table 5.12).[17]
- The width of the narrowest portion (neck or vena contracta) of the jet close to the level of the valve (Table 5.12).
- The approximate size of the intra-atrial portion of a central jet. This gives qualitative confirmation of the more accurate flow acceleration and neck size. Usually this is judged by eye, but in severe regurgitation the jet area is usually >8 cm^2, while in mild it is usually <4 cm^2.[18] *If the jet hugs the wall of the LA, it will stretch out, and its area is then a particularly poor guide to severity.*

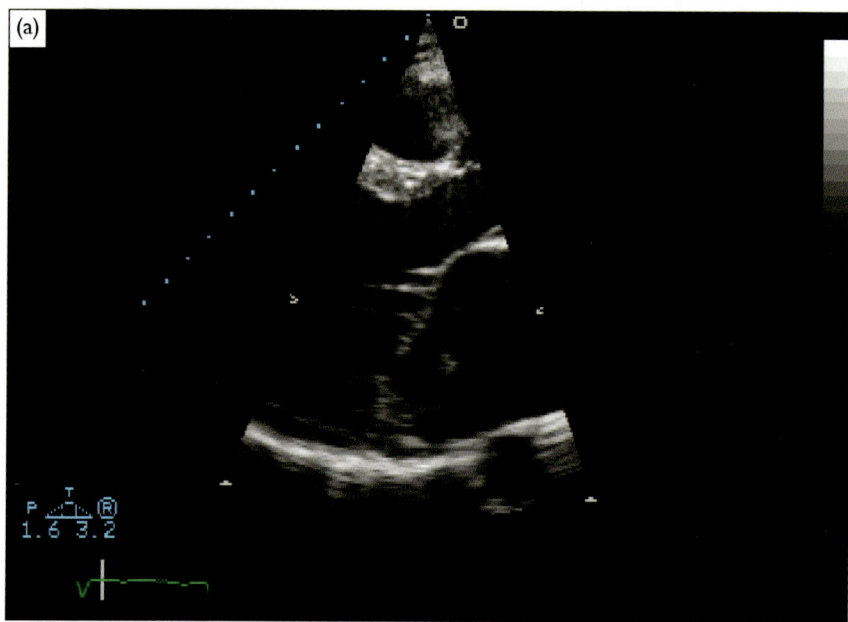

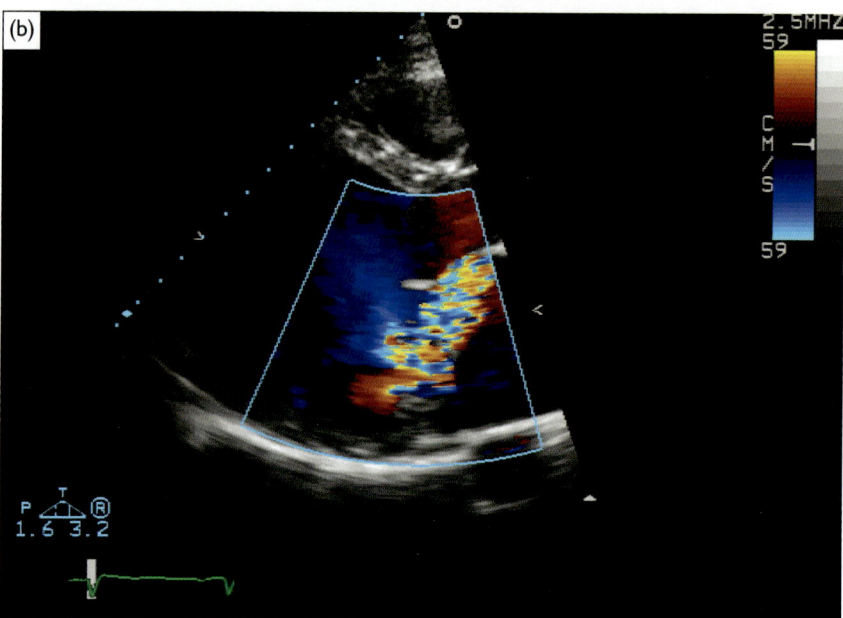

Figure 5.7 Mitral prolapse. The posterior leaflet prolapses (a) and the regurgitant jet is directed anteriorly (b), away from the abnormal leaflet

Valve disease 55

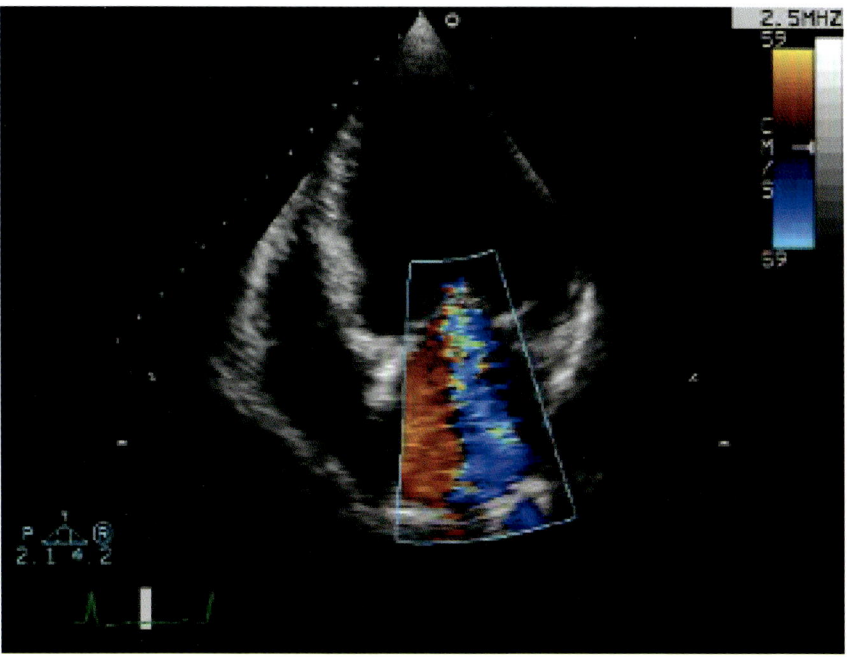

Figure 5.8 Functional mitral regurgitation. In functional regurgitation, as a result of symmetric tenting of the leaflets, the regurgitant jet is central; if one leaflet is slightly more restricted than the other, the jet will be directed towards that leaflet

- The duration of the jet using colour M-mode: Is it holosystolic or present only in part of systole?

3. Continuous-wave signal

- Look at the shape and density of the signal. A signal as dense as forward flow suggests severe regurgitation, a low intensity or incomplete signal mild regurgitation, and an intermediate signal moderate regurgitation.
- Rapid depressurisation of the signal causes a 'dagger-shaped' signal, and is a sign of severe regurgitation.

4. Pulsed Doppler

- A high transmitral E-wave velocity (>1.2 m/s) in the absence of mitral stenosis suggests severe regurgitation.[19]
- A pulsed sample in the pulmonary vein at a distance from the jet can aid quantification, although this is most useful in TOE. Blunting of

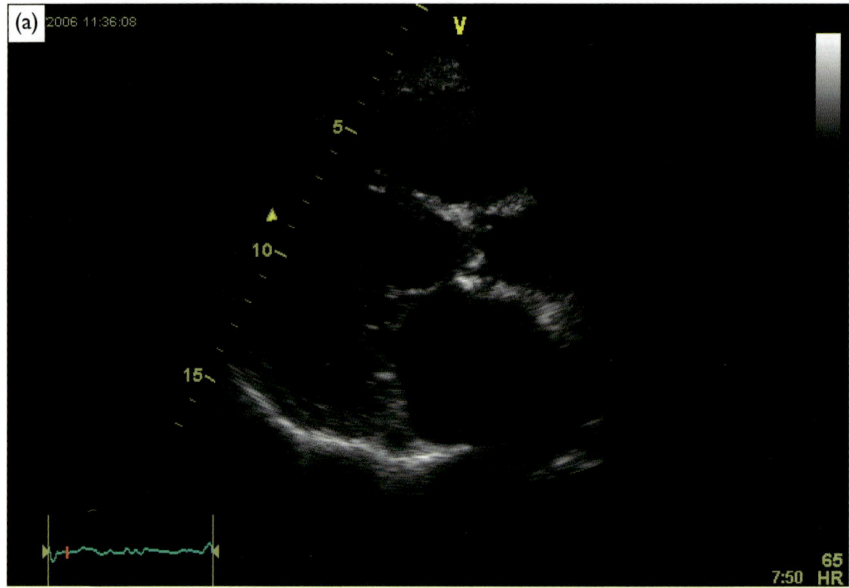
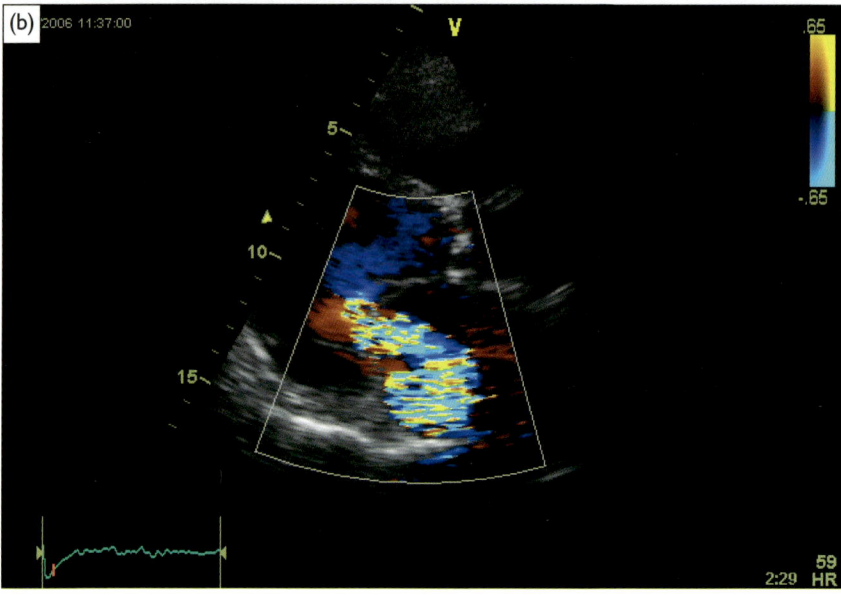

Figure 5.9 Posterior leaflet restriction. In this patient with an inferoposterior myocardial infarction, the posterior leaflet is restricted (a) and the regurgitant jet is directed under the abnormal leaflet (b)

the systolic signal occurs in moderate and severe regurgitation, and flow reversal in very severe regurgitation.

5. Other methods of assessing degree of regurgitation

- A dilated LA is non-specific, but is usual with severe chronic regurgitation.
- A hyperdynamic LV strongly suggests severe regurgitation.
- Moderate pulmonary hypertension (systolic pressure up to 50 mmHg) may complicate severe mitral regurgitation.

6. Grading regurgitation

- *Make a judgement based on all modalities, with the specific signs in Table 5.12 supported by the signal intensity and shape on continuous-wave, LV activity, and pulmonary vein flow pattern.*

7. LV function

- Measure the linear dimensions at the base of the heart and calculate the fractional shortening. The systolic dimension is particularly important, and should be averaged over several measurements. In the absence of a regional wall-motion abnormality, a systolic dimension of 4.0 cm is a threshold for surgery even with no symptoms.
- The LV shape may often change in severe mitral regurgitation, and the LV systolic volume (biplane Simpson's method) aids in the detection of progressive LV dilatation on serial studies.
- *Severe regurgitation causes increased LV activity. Apparently normal systolic function implies myocardial dysfunction.* A fractional shortening <29%, LV ejection fraction <60%, or LV systolic diameter >4.5 cm or end-systolic volume >90 ml/m^2 suggest a relatively low chance of full LV recovery after surgery.

8. Mitral valve repair

- A checklist for suitability for repair before surgery is given in Table 5.13 and one for the assessment after surgery in Table 5.14.
- After repair, it is normal for the posterior leaflet to be echodense and fixed. Most surgeons use an annuloplasty ring in most repairs (Figure 5.9).

Table 5.13 Guide to suitability for repair

Usually repairable by a suitably experienced surgeon
- Posterior prolapse, especially affecting only the middle scallop (P2)
- Localised anterior prolapse
- Perforation
- Localised commissural prolapse
- Localised vegetation without valve destruction
- Mild tenting of the leaflets
- Mild restriction of the posterior leaflet

Repair difficult or impossible
- Widespread involvement of anterior and posterior leaflets
- Rheumatic disease
- Extensive destruction in endocarditis
- Severely restricted posterior leaflet with eccentric jet
- Severe tenting
- Dense annular calcification (debridement risks posterior LV rupture)

Table 5.14 Echocardiography after mitral valve repair

- Appearance of the mitral valve and annuloplasty ring
- Presence, localisation, and grade of residual regurgitation
- Presence and degree of stenosis
- Is there new systolic anterior motion of the anterior leaflet and LV outflow acceleration?
- LV size and function
- RV size and function
- LA size

Checklist for reporting mitral regurgitation

1. Aetiology of mitral regurgitation
2. Detailed description of valve
3. Severity of regurgitation
4. LV dimensions and systolic function
5. PA pressure
6. Other valve disease

TRICUSPID STENOSIS AND REGURGITATION

1. Is the valve morphologically normal?

- *Rheumatic disease is easily missed, since the valve thickening is less marked than on the left. Other causes of organic disease are given in Table 5.15.*
- Is there another cause for regurgitation, such as annular dilatation or a pacing electrode?

Table 5.15 Causes of tricuspid valve disease

- Rheumatic disease (severe thickening uncommon)
- Myxomatous degeneration
- Endocarditis (intravenous drug abuser, Swan–Ganz catheter)
- Carcinoid
- Congenital e.g. Ebstein's anomaly
- Amyloid (general thickening)

2. Grading tricuspid regurgitation

See Table 5.16.

Table 5.16 Grading tricuspid regurgitation[17]

	Mild	Moderate	Severe
Colour neck (mm)	Usually none	<7	>7
PISA radius (cm)^a	<0.5	0.6–0.9	>0.9
Jet area (cm^2)	<5	5–10	>10
Continuous-wave	Incomplete	Low or moderate intensity	Dense and may be triangular (Figure 5.10)
Hepatic vein flow	Normal	Maybe systolic blunting	Systolic reversal (Figure 5.11)

^{a}Colour scale limit 28 cm/s

3. What is the estimated PA pressure?

See page 94.

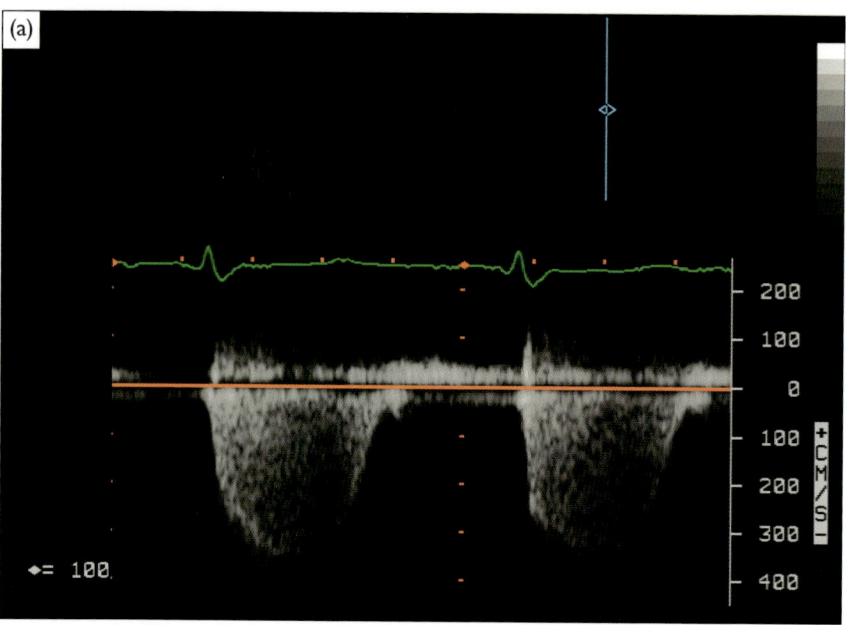

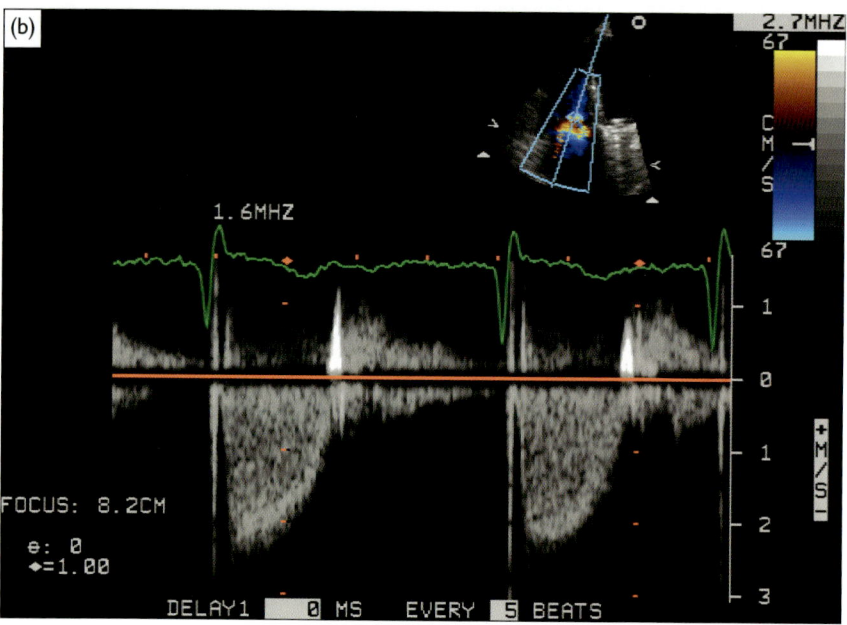

Figure 5.10 Severe tricuspid regurgitation. Moderate or severe regurgitation causes a large intra-atrial jet on colour mapping, with a dense continuous-wave signal that retains its usual shape (a). In torrential regurgitation, the continuous-wave signal (b) may be dagger-shaped.

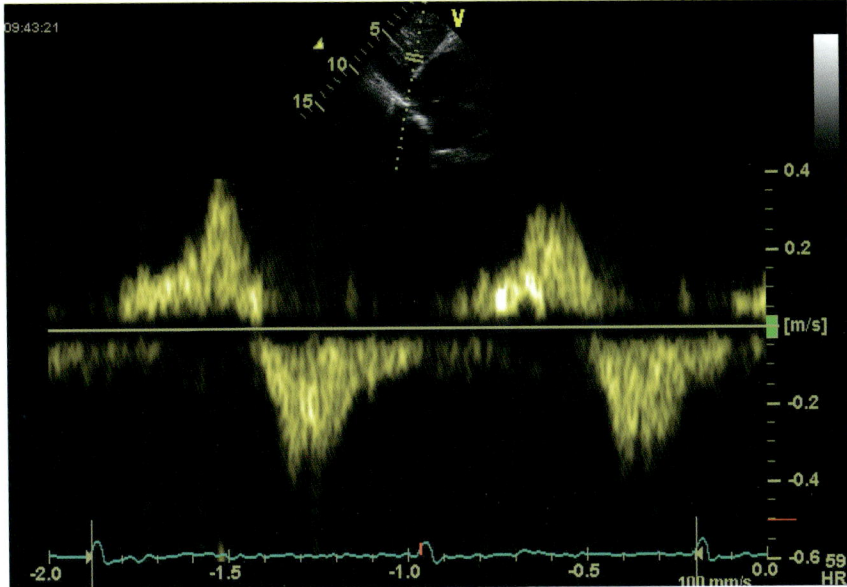

Figure 5.11 Severe tricuspid regurgitation. Flow reversal in a hepatic vein.

4. Is tricuspid stenosis present? (Figure 5.12)

- This is suggested by a $V_{max} > 1$ m/s and is likely if $V_{max} > 1.5$ m/s in the absence of severe tricuspid regurgitation[20] or if the mean gradient is >2 mmHg.[21]
- The pressure half-time is prolonged in severe stenosis, but may vary with respiration and is not reliable.
- Another clue is a small RV (because of underfilling) and a large RA (because of high back-pressure).

PULMONARY STENOSIS AND REGURGITATION

1. Appearance of the valve

- Even in severe stenosis, there may be little thickening, but the valve will be visible in systole as well as diastole.
- The most obvious clue is turbulent high-velocity flow during systole on colour Doppler mapping.

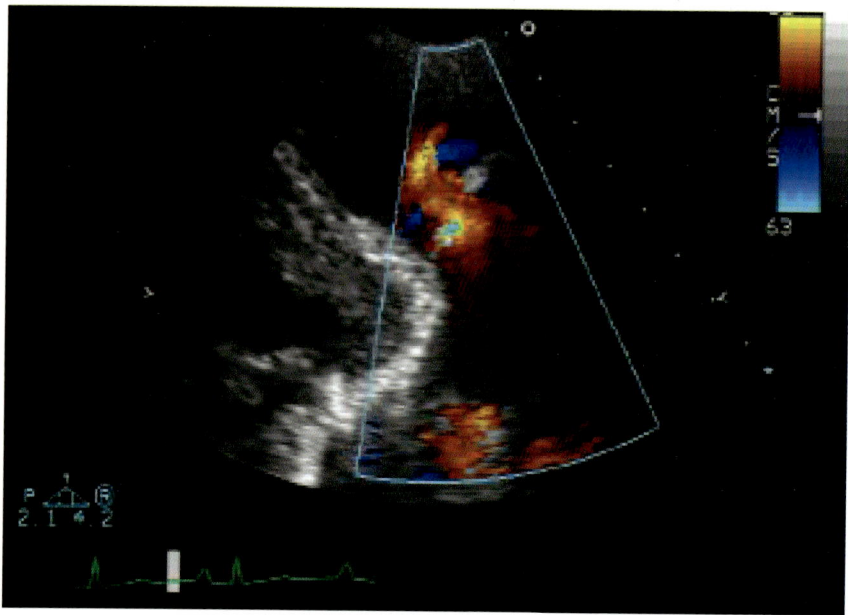

Figure 5.12 Tricuspid stenosis. Tricuspid stenosis may be missed because (unlike the situation with the mitral valve) there is little thickening or calcification.

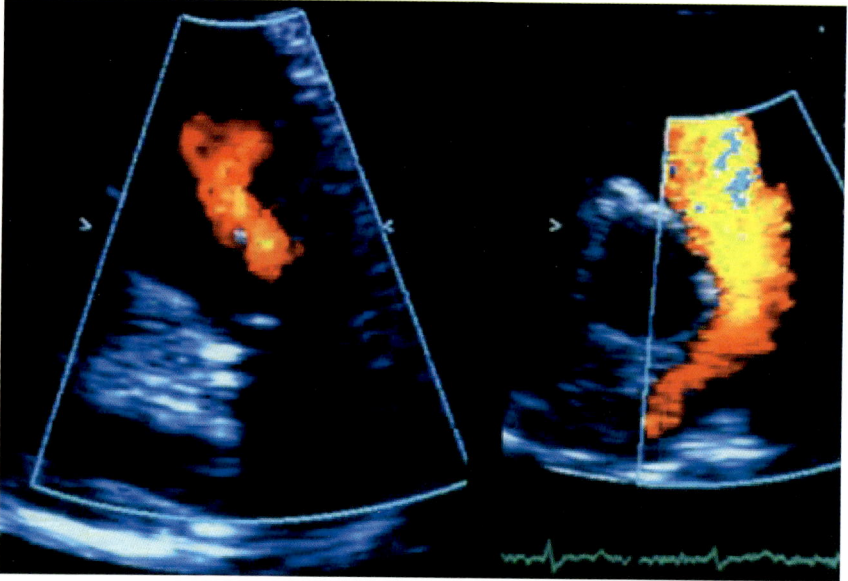

Figure 5.13 Pulmonary regurgitation. Mild regurgitation is shown on the left, with a narrow jet originating at the valve level. Severe regurgitation on the right has a jet filling the RV outflow tract with flow reversal as far as the right PA branch

2. Is pulmonary regurgitation present?

Severe regurgitation is suggested by the following:[22]

- a wide color jet (e.g., >7.5 mm or filling the RV outflow tract)
- diastolic flow reversal visible in the distal main PA (Figure 5.13)
- a steep dense signal (pressure half-time <100 ms)
- active dilated RV.

3. What is the pressure difference across the valve?

Severe stenosis is suggested by the following:[2,23]

- transpulmonary V_{max} >4 m/s
- mean pressure difference >50 mmHg
- mean pressure difference <50 mmHg with RV dysfunction.

4. What is the pulmonary artery pressure? See page 94

- Dominant pulmonary regurgitation may be caused by pulmonary hypertension.
- Pulmonary stenosis tends to protect the pulmonary circulation against the effect of high flow from a left-to-right shunt.

REFERENCES

1. Kennedy KD, Nishimura RA, Holmes DR Jr, Bailey KR. Natural history of moderate aortic stenosis. J Am Coll Cardiol 1991; 17:313–19.
2. Bonow RO et al. ACC/AHA 2006 guidelines for the management of patients with valvular heart disease: a report of the American College of Cardiology/American Heart Association Task Force on Practice Guidelines. J Am Coll Cardiol 2006; 48:e1–148.
3. Monin JL, Quere JP, Monchi M, et al. Low-gradient aortic stenosis: operative risk stratification and predictors for long-term outcome: a multicenter study using dobutamine stress hemodynamics. Circulation 2003; 108:319–24.
4. Chambers J. Low 'gradient', low flow aortic stenosis. Heart 2006; 92:554–8.
5. Nishimura RA, Grantham JA, Connolly HM, et al. Low-output, low-gradient aortic stenosis in patients with depressed left ventricular systolic function: the clinical utility of the dobutamine challenge in the catheterization laboratory. Circulation 2002; 106:809–13.
6. Iung B, Gohlke-Barwolf C, Tornos P, Tribouilloy C, et al. Recommendations on the management of the asymptomatic patient with valvular heart disease. Eur Heart J 2002; 23:1252–66.
7. Dujardin KS, Enriquez-Sarano M, Schaff HV, et al. Mortality and morbidity of aortic regurgitation in clinical practice. A long-term follow-up study. Circulation 1999; 99:1851–7.
8. Perry GJ, Helmcke F, Nanda NC, Byard C, Soto B. Evaluation of aortic insufficiency by Doppler color flow mapping. J Am Coll Cardiol 1987; 9:952–9.
9. Teague SM, Heinsimer JA, Anderson JL, et al. Quantification of aortic regurgitation utilizing continuous wave Doppler ultrasound. J Am Coll Cardiol 1986; 8:592–9.

10. Samstad SO, Hegrenaes L, Skjaerpe T, Hatle L. Half time of the diastolic aortoventricular pressure difference by continuous wave Doppler ultrasound: a measure of the severity of aortic regurgitation? Br Heart J 1989; 61:336–43.
11. Willett DL, Hall SA, Jessen ME, Wait MA, Grayburn PA. Assessment of aortic regurgitation by transesophageal color Doppler imaging of the vena contracta: validation against an intraoperative aortic flow probe. J Am Coll Cardiol 2001; 37:1450–5.
12. Tribouilloy C, Avinee P, Shen WF, et al. End diastolic flow velocity just beneath the aortic isthmus assessed by pulsed Doppler echocardiography: a new predictor of the aortic regurgitant fraction. Br Heart J 1991; 65:37–40.
13. Bonow RO, Carabello B, de LA Jr, et al. Guidelines for the management of patients with valvular heart disease: executive summary. A report of the American College of Cardiology/American Heart Association Task Force on Practice Guidelines (Committee on Management of Patients with Valvular Heart Disease). Circulation 1998; 98:1949–84.
14. Reid CL, Otto CM, Davis KB, et al. Influence of mitral valve morphology on mitral balloon commissurotomy: immediate and six-month results from the NHLBI Balloon Valvuloplasty Registry. Am Heart J 1992; 124:657–65.
15. Fawzy ME, Hegazy H, Shoukri M, et al. Long-term clinical and echocardiographic results after successful mitral balloon valvotomy and predictors of long-term outcome. Eur Heart J 2005; 26:1647–52.
16. Wilkins GT, Weyman AE, Abascal VM, Block PC, Palacios IF. Percutaneous balloon dilatation of the mitral valve: an analysis of echocardiographic variables related to outcome and the mechanism of dilatation. Br Heart J 1988; 60:299–308.
17. Zoghbi WA, Enriquez-Sarano M, Foster E, et al. Recommendations for evaluation of the severity of native valvular regurgitation with two-dimensional and Doppler echocardiography. J Am Soc Echocardiogr 2003; 16:777–802.
18. Spain MG, Smith MD, Grayburn PA, Harlamert EA, DeMaria AN. Quantitative assessment of mitral regurgitation by Doppler color flow imaging: angiographic and hemodynamic correlations. J Am Coll Cardiol 1989; 13:585–90.
19. Thomas L, Foster E, Schiller NB. Peak mitral inflow velocity predicts mitral regurgitation severity. J Am Coll Cardiol 1998; 31:174–9.
20. Parris TM, Panidis JP, Ross J, Mintz GS. Doppler echocardiographic findings in rheumatic tricuspid stenosis. Am J Cardiol 1987; 60:1414–16.
21. Ribeiro PA, Al Zaibag M, Al Kasab S, et al. Provocation and amplification of the transvalvular pressure gradient in rheumatic tricuspid stenosis. Am J Cardiol 1988; 61:1307–11.
22. Rodriguez RJ, Riggs TW. Physiologic peripheral pulmonic stenosis in infancy. Am J Cardiol 1990; 66:1478–81.
23. Silvilairat S, Cabalka AK, Cetta F, Hagler DJ, O'Leary PW. Echocardiographic assessment of isolated pulmonary valve stenosis: Which outpatient Doppler gradient has the most clinical validity? J Am Soc Echocardiogr 2005; 18:1137–42.

6 PROSTHETIC VALVES

GENERAL

- All prosthetic valves are obstructive compared with a normal native valve, and it is important to differentiate normal from pathologic obstruction.
- Minor regurgitation through the valve is usually normal, and the pattern differs between the types.

1. Appearance of the valve

- Note the position and type (Figure 6.1 and Table 6.1).

Table 6.1 Types of replacement heart valve (see also Appendix 2)

Biological
Stented xenograft
- Porcine
- Pericardial

Stentless
- Autograft
- Homograft
- Porcine xenograft
- Pericardial xenograft

Mechanical
- Caged-ball
- Tilting disc
- Bileaflet

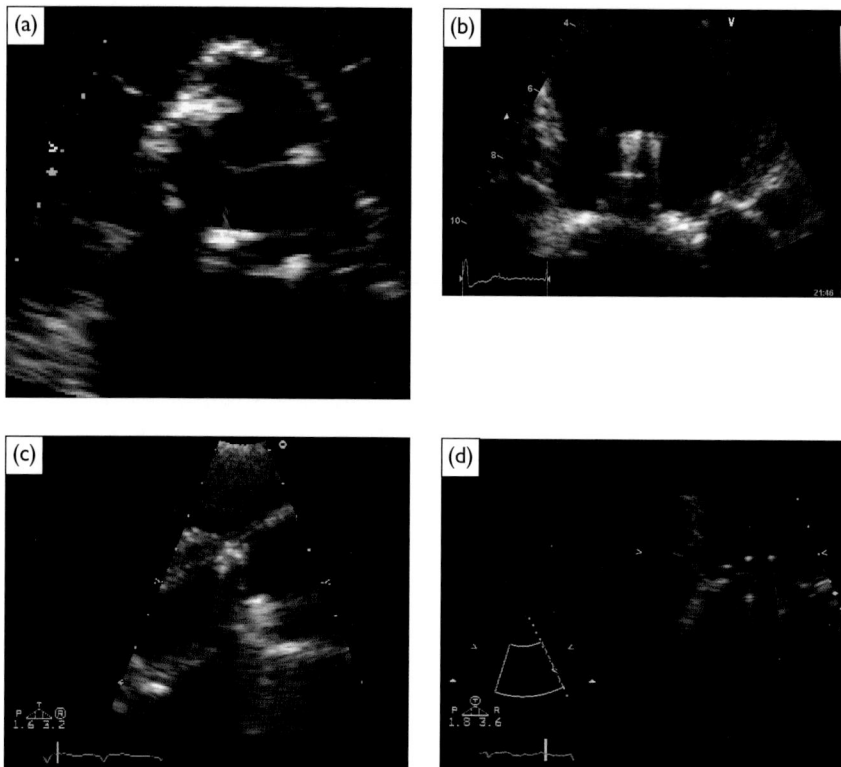

Figure 6.1 Echocardiograms of prosthetic heart valves. (a) Stented porcine aortic xenograft in a parasternal short-axis view. (b) Caged-ball mitral valve in a 4-chamber view. (c) Tilting-disk aortic valve in a parasternal long-axis view. (d) Zoomed view of a bileaflet mechanical mitral valve in a 4-chamber view

- Does the prosthesis rock? In the aortic position, this is always caused by a large dehiscence (usually >30% of the sewing ring). In the mitral position, it may be as a result of conservation of the native leaflets.

If the valve is biological

- Are the cusps thickened (>3 mm in thickness)?
- Is cusp motion normal, or is there decreased motion (suggesting obstruction) or increased motion (suggesting a tear). Increased motion can either be due to prolapse or a flail cusp or segment (moving through 180°).
- Newly implanted (up to 6 months) stentless valves may be associated with a thickened aortic root caused by oedema and haematoma.

Occasionally, this may be mistaken for an abscess on transoesophageal echocardiography.
- Is there a separate echogenic mass (either vegetation or torn cusp).

If the valve is mechanical
- Does the occluder (disk or ball or leaflets) open quickly and fully?
- If there are two leaflets, does each open and close symmetrically?
  - Minor variation in closing time may occasionally be seen in a mitral valve.
  - Fluttering of the leaflets of a bileaflet valve is normal.
- Is there a separate echogenic mass attached to the valve?
  - Consider thrombus or a vegetation.
  - If thin, it could be a fibrin strand, which is normal.
- Dense spontaneous echoes in the LV cavity are normal in replacement mitral mechanical valves.

2. Is there regurgitation or evidence of obstruction?
- Interpretation depends on the position of the valve (pages 67–73).

3. LV and RV function and PA pressure
- A hyperdynamic LV is a clue that there is severe prosthetic aortic or mitral regurgitation. A hyperdynamic RV suggests severe right-sided prosthetic regurgitation.
- A rise in PA pressure can be a sign of prosthetic mitral valve obstruction.

4. When is TOE needed? (Table 6.2)
- TTE and TOE are complementary and TOE is rarely used without initial TTE. Although the transoesophageal approach is usually necessary to image vegetations and posterior root abscesses, anterior root abscesses may be better seen on TTE.

AORTIC POSITION

1. Is there any regurgitation?
- How many jets and where are they?
  - The site of an aortic jet can be described on the sewing ring as a clockface in the parasternal short-axis view.

Table 6.2 Indications for TOE

- Endocarditis at least a moderate possibility
- Obstruction of a mechanical valve to determine the cause (Table 6.3)
- Obstruction not certain (equivocal EOA and cusp or occluder poorly imaged transthoracically)
- Abnormal regurgitation suspected, but transthoracic study normal or equivocal:
  – Breathless patient
  – Hyperdynamic LV
  – Haemolysis
- Mitral regurgitant jet of uncertain size
- Thromboembolism despite adequate anticoagulation (look for pannus or thrombus)

- Is the regurgitation through the valve, paraprosthetic, or both? Localisation can only be certain if:
  – the base or neck of the jet can be imaged in relation to the sewing ring (Figure 6.2) or
  – for a mechanical valve, the study matches the typical pattern of normal regurgitation (Figure 6.3)
- *Regurgitation through the valve in bileaflet mechanical valves ('pivotal washing jets') begins close to the edge of the orifice and must not be mistaken for paraprosthetic jets.*
- Is it normal or abnormal?
  – Mild regurgitation is commonly seen through biological valves and is usually normal. However, when associated with a thickened cusp, it is an early sign of primary failure – especially if it increases on serial studies.
  – Normal regurgitation through a mechanical valve is usually low in momentum (relatively homogeneous colour), with an incomplete or very low-intensity continuous-wave signal.

2. Severity of regurgitation

- Use the same methods as for native regurgitation (see page 46). Assessing the height of a jet relative to LV outflow diameter may be difficult, since paraprosthetic jets are often eccentric.
- The circumference of the sewing ring occupied by the aortic jet is another guide: mild (<10%), moderate (10–20%), severe (>20%).

Table 6.3 Causes of obstruction in a mechanical valve

- Thrombosis
- Pannus
- Vegetations
- Mechanical (e.g. chord, septal bulge)

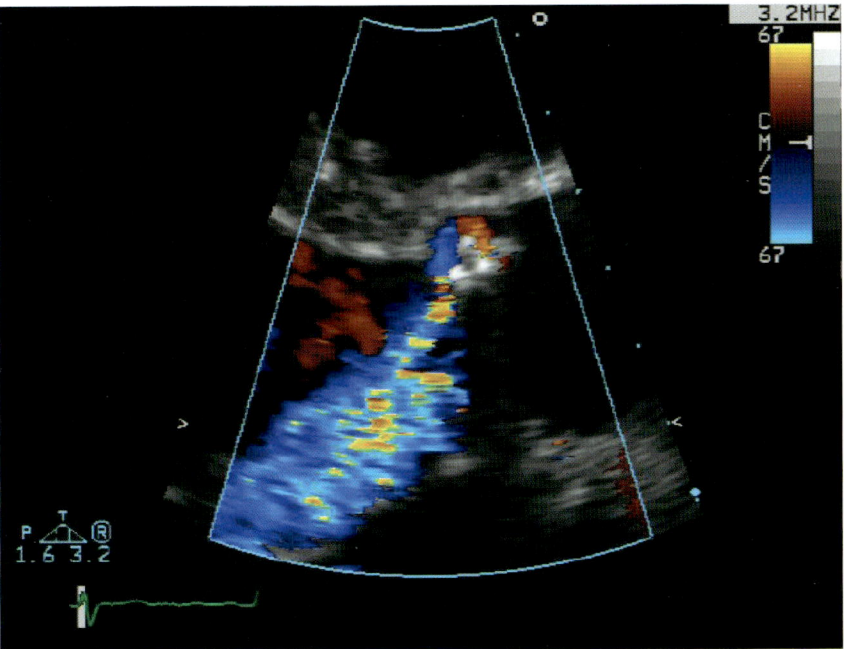

Figure 6.2 Paraprosthetic regurgitation. Parasternal long-axis view of a bileaflet mechanical aortic valve. There is a jet originating in the aorta, with the neck clearly imaged outside the sewing ring and directed eccentrically in the LV outflow tract

3. Is there evidence of obstruction? (Table 6.4)

- In biological valves, this is shown by thickened and immobile cusps. The disk or leaflets of an obstructed mechanical valve may be difficult to image even on TOE, but obstruction in mechanical valves in the aortic position is rare.
- Measure V_{max} and peak and mean gradient, and EOA using the classical form of the continuity equation. Compare with normal values for type and size (Appendix 2).

Table 6.4 When to suspect aortic obstruction

> - Thickened or immobile cusps or occluder
> - Measurements outside normal values (see Appendix 2)
> - Change in measurements by about 25% on serial studies

- TOE is occasionally necessary to confirm normal leaflet motion in a valve with an equivocal EOA.

MITRAL POSITION

1. Is there regurgitation?

- An easily seen jet is usually paraprosthetic, since normal transprosthetic regurgitation tends to be hidden by flow shielding (unless the LA is very large).
- The intraventricular flow recruitment region of a paraprosthetic regurgitant jet can usually be seen even when the intra-atrial jet is invisible. This allows the regurgitation to be localised using the sewing-ring as a clockface.

2. Severity of mitral prosthetic regurgitation

- Severe paraprosthetic regurgitation may be obvious from:
  - a large region of flow acceleration within the LV
  - a broad neck
  - a hyperdynamic LV
  - a dense continuous-wave signal, especially with early depressurisation (dagger shape).
- If there is doubt, TOE is necessary to evaluate jet width, the size of the intra-atrial jet, and PV flow (looking for systolic flow reversal).

3. Is there evidence of obstruction? (Table 6.5)

- Most information for the diagnosis of obstruction is found from imaging and colour flow mapping.
- Measure V_{max} and mean gradient, and compare with normal values (Appendix 2).
- *Pressure half-time does not reflect orifice area in normally functioning prosthetic mitral valves so the Hatle orifice area formula is not*

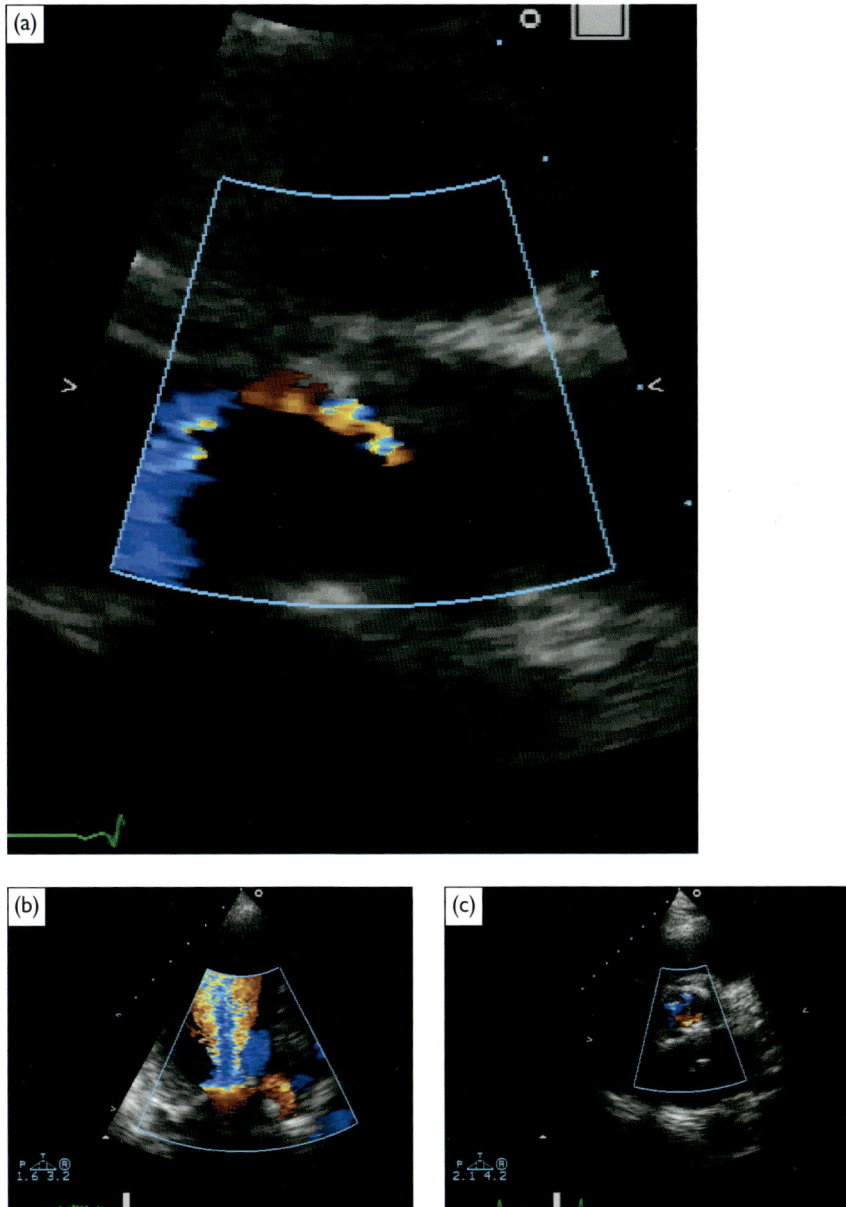

Figure 6.3 Normal transprosthetic regurgitation. (a) A thin jet of regurgitation through a homograft aortic valve imaged in a parasternal long-axis view. (b) A tilting-disk aortic valve imaged in an apical long-axis view, showing regurgitation related to the major and minor orifices. (c) A bileaflet mechanical aortic valve in a parasternal short-axis view, showing two jets from the upper and two from the lower pivotal point

Table 6.5 When to suspect mitral obstruction

- Thickened and immobile cusps or occluder
- Narrowed colour inflow
- Pressure half-time >200 ms with V_{max} >2.5 m/s
- Change in measurements by about 25% from previous study
- Increase in PA pressure

valid. However, the pressure half-time lengthens significantly when the valve becomes obstructed.

RIGHT-SIDED

- Tricuspid annuloplasty is performed if there is more than moderate tricuspid regurgitation in the presence of left-sided disease. Tricuspid replacement valves are not often implanted, and pulmonary replacements are even less common.

1. Is there regurgitation?

- Regurgitation is easily seen after implantation of an annuloplasty ring or with a pulmonary replacement.
- Tricuspid regurgitation may be partially shielded. Use multiple views and look for flow reversal in the hepatic vein and a hyperdynamic RV.

2. Severity of regurgitation

- This is as for native tricuspid and pulmonary regurgitation.

Table 6.6 When to suspect tricuspid obstruction[1,2]

- Thickened and immobile cusps or occluder
- Narrowed colour inflow
- Dilated IVC or RA
- Peak velocity >1.5 m/s (in the absence of severe tricuspid regurgitation)
- Mean gradient >5 mmHg
- Pressure half-time >240 ms

3. Is there evidence of obstruction?

- Because of respiratory variability, measurements should be made over several cycles for the tricuspid valve even if in sinus rhythm (Tables 6.6 and 6.7).

Table 6.7 When to suspect pulmonary obstruction[3]

- Cusp thickening or immobility
- Narrowing of colour flow
- V_{max} >3 m/s (suspicious, not diagnostic)
- Increase in peak velocity on serial studies (more reliable)
- Impaired RV function

Checklist for reporting prosthetic valves
1. Valve position and type
2. Doppler forward flow values
3. LV dimensions and function (RV function for right-sided valves)
4. Pulmonary artery pressure
5. Any signs of obstruction?
6. Regurgitation: site and degree

REFERENCES

1. Connolly HM, Miller FA Jr, Taylor CL, et al. Doppler hemodynamic profiles of 82 clinically and echocardiographically normal tricuspid valve prostheses. Circulation 1993; 88:2722–7.
2. Kobayashi Y, Nagata S, Ohmori F, et al. Serial doppler echocardiographic evaluation of bioprosthetic valves in the tricuspid position. J Am Coll Cardiol 1996; 27:1693–7.
3. Novaro GM, Connolly HM, Miller FA. Doppler hemodynamics of 51 clinically and echocardiographically normal pulmonary valve prostheses. Mayo Clin Proc 2001; 76:155–60.

7 ENDOCARDITIS

The echocardiographic signs of endocarditis are as follows:

- vegetation
- local complication (Table 7.1)
- valve destruction.

Table 7.1 Local complications of endocarditis

- Abscess (Figure 7.1)
- Fistula
- Perforation
- Aneurysm of a leaflet
- Dehiscence of a replacement valve

1. Is there a vegetation?

- This is typically a mass attached to the valve and moving with a different phase to the leaflet.
- *However, sometimes it may be difficult to differentiate from other types of masses (e.g. calcific or myxomatous degeneration). A term should be chosen that will not lead to overdiagnosis of endocarditis (Table 7.2).*
- Note the size and mobility of the vegetation. Highly mobile masses larger than 10 mm in length[1] have a relatively high risk of embolisation and may affect the decision for surgery.

2. Is there a local complication? (Table 7.1)

- A new paraprosthetic leak is a reliable sign of prosthetic endocarditis provided there is a baseline postoperative study showing no leak.

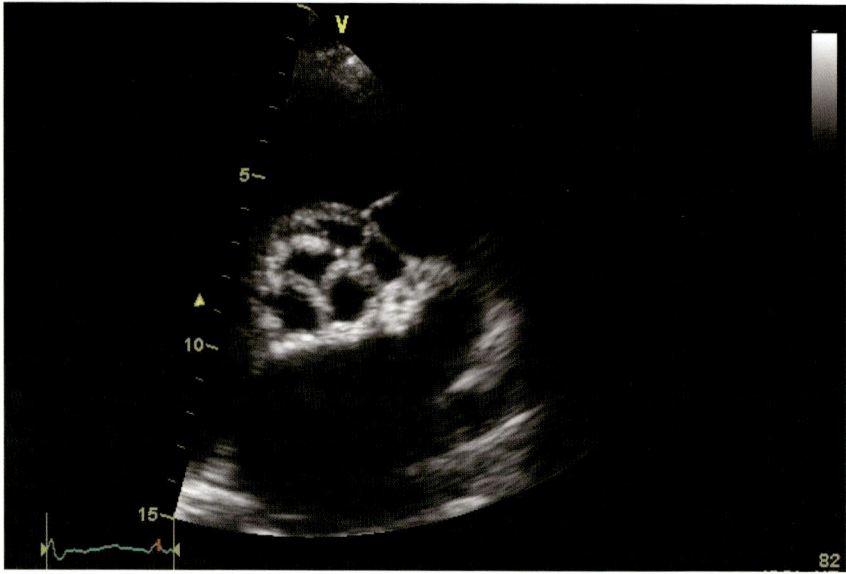

Figure 7.1 Aortic abscess. Parasternal short-axis view showing cavities between the PA and aorta and in the anterior aorta. The aortic valve cusps are thickened because of endocarditis

Table 7.2 Terms suitable for describing a mass

- 'Typical of a vegetation'
- 'Consistent with a vegetation'
- 'Consistent but not diagnostic of a vegetation'
- 'Consistent with a vegetation but more in keeping with calcific degeneration'
- 'Most consistent with calcific degeneration'

- An abscess usually suggests that surgery will be necessary.

3. Is there valve destruction?

- New or worsening regurgitation is a sign of endocarditis, even if no vegetation is visible.
- Disruption of the edges of a cusp suggests endocarditis.
- Severe or progressive regurgitation suggest the need for early surgery.

4. Assess the LV

- Progressive systolic dilatation of the LV is one criterion for surgery.
- *If there is acute severe aortic regurgitation, look for signs of a raised LV end-diastolic pressure as an indication for urgent surgery:*
    - on M-mode, closure of the mitral valve at or before the Q wave
    - on transmitral pulsed Doppler, an E deceleration time <150 ms
    - diastolic mitral regurgitation.

5. Assess predisposing abnormality

See Table 7.3.

Table 7.3 Predisposing abnormalities

- Valve disease
- Replacement heart valves
- Congenital disease (other than ASD)
- Hypertrophic cardiomyopathy

6. Is TOE necessary?

See Table 7.4.

Table 7.4 Indications for TOE in endocarditis

- Prosthetic valve
- Pacemaker
- Suspicion of abscess on transthoracic study
- Normal or equivocal TTE and continuing clinical suspicion of endocarditis

---

Checklist for reporting endocarditis

1. Is there a vegetation, local complication, or evidence of valve destruction?
2. Grade of regurgitation?
3. Severity of predisposing disease (e.g., valve stenosis or VSD)
4. LV dimensions and function (or RV for tricuspid valve endocarditis)

REFERENCE

1. Thuny F, Disalvo G, Belliard O, et al. Risk of embolism and death in infective endocarditis: prognostic value of echocardiography: a prospective multicenter study. Circulation 2005; 112:69–75.

8 AORTA

- The ascending thoracic aorta should be examined if the initial minimum standard study shows:
  - aortic dilatation
  - significant aortic stenosis or regurgitation
  - a bicuspid aortic valve.
- The whole of the thoracic aorta and also the abdominal aorta should be examined in patients with:
  - suspected aortic dissection (usually using TOE)
  - a predisposition to aortic dilatation (e.g., Marfan syndrome, Ehlers–Danlos syndrome type IV)
  - a widened mediastinum on the chest X-ray
  - trauma (usually using TOE).

AORTIC DILATATION

1. What is the diameter of the aorta?

- Measure the diameter at all levels (Figure 8.1) and compare with normal ranges (Table 8.1).
- Aortic size is related to body habitus and age (Table 8.1); and see Figures A1.3 and A1.4 in Appendix 1).
- A sinotubular junction diameter greater than the annulus diameter by around 20% suggests early dilatation, even if the absolute values are normal.
- Typical dilatation in Marfan syndrome affects predominantly annulus and sinuses, causing a 'pear-shaped' aorta. Arteriosclerotic dilatation typically affects the ascending aorta.
- Minimum thresholds for referral for surgery are given (Table 8.2).

Table 8.1 Normal ranges for aortic diameter (cm)[1-5]

Site	Range	Indexed to BSA
A Annulus	1.7–2.5	1.1–1.5
B Sinus of Valsalva	2.2–3.6	1.4–2.1
C Sinotubular junction	1.8–2.6	1.0–1.6
D Ascending	2.1–3.4	
E Arch	1.4–2.9	0.8–1.9
F Descending	1.1–2.3	0.8–1.2
G Abdominal	1.0–2.2	0.6–1.3

Table 8.2 Thresholds for considering surgical referral in aortic dilatation

Arteriosclerotic dilatation	5.5 cm[a,6]
Marfan and Ehlers–Danlos syndromes	4.5 cm[a,6,7]
Bicuspid valve	5.0 cm (or 2.5 cm/m^2)[8]
Bicuspid valve if aortic valve replacement is independently indicated	4.5 cm[8]
The maximum diameter is used, regardless of level	

[a]Some recommend surgery at 6 cm in arteriosclerotic dilatation and 5.5 cm in Marfan syndrome. Lower thresholds assume a young fit subject and a specialist surgical team with excellent results. The decision for surgery also depends on the rate of increase in diameter and on clinical factors.

2. How much aortic regurgitation?

See page 46.

3. Check for coarctation

- If there is a bicuspid aortic valve or unexplained aortic dilatation in a young subject.

BEFORE AORTIC VALVE SURGERY

1. Dimensions of ascending aorta

See Table 8.1: A–D.

Aorta

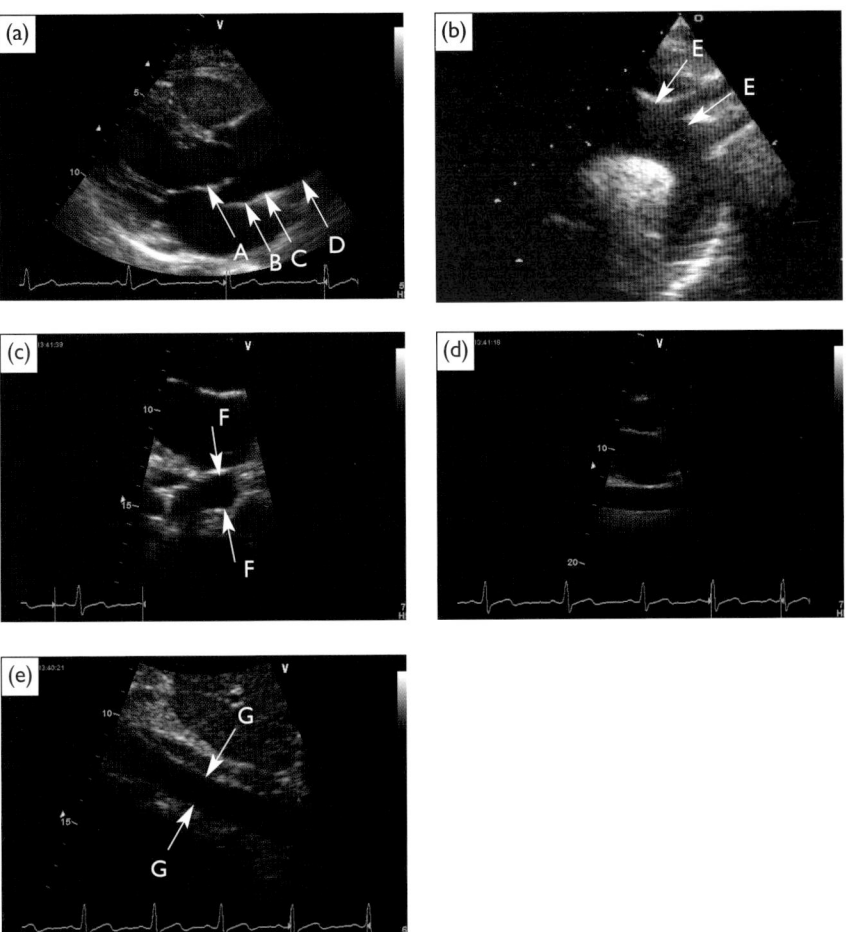

Figure 8.1 Levels for measuring the diameter of the aorta. Many normal ranges are based on measurements taken from leading edge to leading edge, while current guidelines for assessment recommend measuring from inner edge to inner edge. Errors based on this discrepancy are likely to be small. (a) Parasternal long-axis view of the annulus (level A in Table 8.1), sinus (level B), sinotubular junction (level C), and ascending aorta (level D). (b) Suprasternal view of the arch (level E) (two possible measurement sites). (c) Parasternal long-axis view showing the descending thoracic aorta (level F) in short-axis. (d) Rotated view to show the descending thoracic aorta in long-axis. (e) Abdominal aorta (level G) in a subcostal view

2. Is there significant calcification in the aorta?

- Severe calcification may preclude implanting a stentless valve, may affect the site of the trochars for the bypass machine, and may occasionally preclude aortic valve replacement altogether.

DISSECTION

1. Is there a dissection flap?

- An intraluminal flap is the hallmark of dissection. Blooming from calcium deposits or reverberation artifact can sometimes cause confusion.
- TTE has limited diagnostic power in dissection. If the study is normal, TOE is always necessary if the clinical suspicion is high (Table 8.3).
- Even if TOE is needed to delineate an intrathoracic flap, a transthoracic study is better at showing the distal extent of the dissection in the abdominal aorta.

Table 8.3 Role of TOE in suspected dissection

- Detection of dissection flap
- Detection of mural haematoma
- Aortic diameters
- Entry tear
- Involvement of head and neck vessels
- Thrombosis of false lumen

2. What is the maximum aortic diameter?

3. How much aortic regurgitation?

4. Is there pericardial fluid?

- This suggests rupture into the pericardial sac, which is a common cause of death in acute dissection. It may suggest the diagnosis even if a flap cannot be imaged.

5. LV function

- Impaired LV function on TTE can guide the decision for conservative management, especially in dissections involving only the descending thoracic aorta.

MARFAN AND EHLERS–DANLOS SYNDROMES

1. Aortic diameters at all levels

See Table 8.1: A–G.

2. How much aortic regurgitation?

3. Is there mitral or tricuspid prolapse or mitral annulus calcification?

4. Is there coexistent PA dilatation?

See Table 8.4.

Table 8.4 Normal PA dimensions[1]

RV outflow diameter	1.8–3.4 cm
Pulmonary valve annulus	1.0–2.2 cm
Main PA	0.9–2.9 cm
Right pulmonary branch	0.7–1.7 cm
Left pulmonary branch	0.6–1.4 cm

COARCTATION

1. Describe the coarctation

- From the suprasternal position, describe the site in relation to the left subclavian artery and appearance (membrane, tunnel) using imaging and colour flow.
- Measure the aortic dimensions above and below the coarctation.

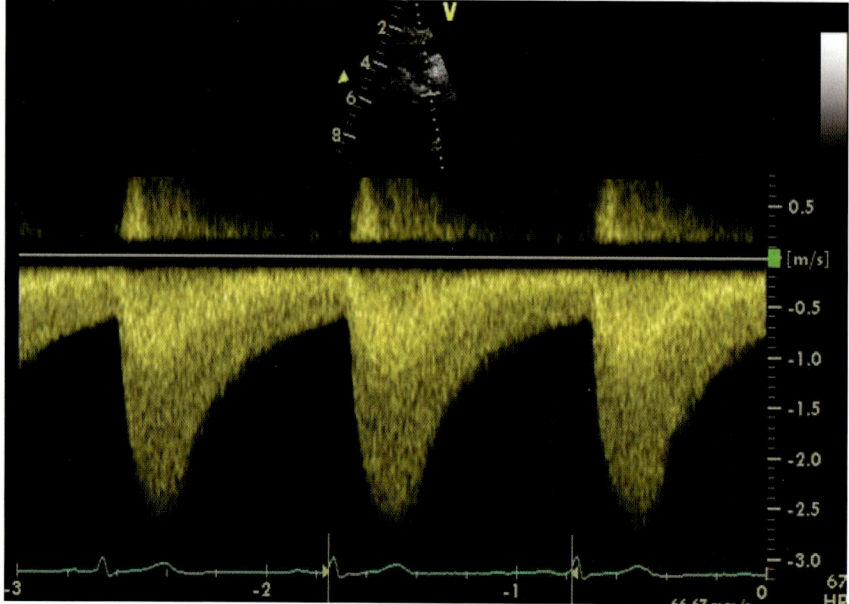

Figure 8.2 Coarctation. Continuous-wave recording from the suprasternal notch

Checklist for reporting the aorta

1. Diameter at each level
2. Aortic regurgitation

Marfan and Ehlers–Danlos syndromes
1, 2, and
3. Mitral (and tricuspid) prolapse and annular calcification
4. PA diameter

Suspected dissection
1, 2, and
5. Dissection flap
6. Pericardial effusion

Coarctation
7. Site
8. Peak velocity
9. Aortic diameter above and below the coarctation and in the ascending aorta
10. Check for bicuspid aortic valve and associated LV hypertrophy

2. Continuous-wave recording

- The most reliable feature on continuous-wave recording is forward flow during diastole (Figure 8.2). Elevated flow velocities are usually seen in systole, but may occasionally be absent or difficult to record if there is a severe or complete coarctation with extensive collaterals. Measure the peak velocity.

3. General

- Look for associated aortic root dilatation and bicuspid aortic valve.
- Check LV mass and LV function.

REFERENCES

1. Triulzi MO, Gillam LD, Gentile F. Normal adult cross-sectional echocardiographic values: linear dimensions and chamber areas. Echocardiography 1984; 1:403–26.
2. Davidson WR Jr, Pasquale MJ, Fanelli C. A Doppler echocardiographic examination of the normal aortic valve and left ventricular outflow tract. Am J Cardiol 1991; 67:547–9.
3. Unpublished work. Guy's Hospital London. Guy's Database, 1995.
4. Mintz GS, Kotler MN, Segal BL, Parry WR. Two dimensional echocardiographic recognition of the descending thoracic aorta. Am J Cardiol 1979; 44:232–8.
5. Schnittger I, Gordon EP, Fitzgerald PJ, Popp RL. Standardized intracardiac measurements of two-dimensional echocardiography. J Am Coll Cardiol 1983; 2:934–8.
6. Elefteriades JA. Natural history of thoracic aortic aneurysms: indications for surgery, and surgical versus nonsurgical risks. Ann Thorac Surg 2002; 74(5):S1877–80; discussion S1892–8.
7. Ergin MA, Spielvogel D, Apaydin A, et al. Surgical treatment of the dilated ascending aorta: when and how? Ann Thorac Surg 1999; 67:1834–9; discussion 1853–6.
8. Bonow RO, et al. ACC/AHA 2006 guidelines for the management of patients with valvular heart disease: a report of the American College of Cardiology/American Heart Association Task Force on Practice Guidelines. J Am Coll Cardiol 2006; 48:e1–148.
9. Erbel R, Alfonso F, Boileau C, et al. Diagnosis and management of aortic dissection. Eur Heart J 2001; 22:1642–81.

9 ATRIA

- A single LA diameter measurement is still recorded in routine clinical practice using 2D, usually in a parasternal long-axis view. Normal is <4.0 cm.
- LA geometry varies, and is not accurately represented by a linear dimension. LA size needs to be assessed more accurately if there is:
  - atrial dilatation noted on the initial study
  - hypertension (as a sign of increased filling pressure)
  - atrial fibrillation (likely success of cardioversion, thromboembolic risk)
  - mitral valve disease (thromboembolic risk, indirect marker of severity).
- A simple clinical method is planimetry of the area in a 4-chamber view, modified if necessary to optimise atrial size (Table 9.1) and frozen at maximum size just before mitral valve opening. For research studies, biplane Simpson's or area–length rule using 4-chamber and 2-chamber views should be indexed to BSA.

Table 9.1 LA dilatation[1,2]

	Mild[a]	Moderate	Severe
LA area (cm^2)	20–29	30–40	>40
LA volume/BSA (ml/m^2)	29–31	32–39	>40

[a]Interpret within the whole echocardiographic and clinical context

- Atrial dilatation can give a clue to the diagnosis (Tables 9.2 and 9.3). A guide threshold for RA dilatation is a transverse diameter >5 cm in the 4-chamber view.

Table 9.2 Causes of severe biatrial enlargement

- Apical hypertrophic cardiomyopathy
- Restrictive cardiomyopathy
- Rheumatic disease affecting mitral and tricuspid valves

Table 9.3 Causes of right atrial dilatation

- Tricuspid stenosis or regurgitation
- Pulmonary hypertension
- ASD
- RV myopathy

REFERENCES

1. Lang RM, Bierig M, Devereux RB, et al. Recommendations for chamber quantification. Eur J Echocardiogr 2006; 7:79–108.
2. Abhayaratna WP, Seward JB, Appleton CP, et al. Left atrial size: physiologic determinants and clinical applications. J Am Coll Cardiol 2006; 47:2357–63.

10 RIGHT HEART

RIGHT VENTRICLE

RV size and function must always be assessed especially if there is:

- RV dilatation on the minimum standard study
- congenital heart disease
- left-sided disease, especially mitral stenosis or severe aortic stenosis
- suspected RV cardiomyopathy
- pulmonary hypertension
- suspected pulmonary embolism
- chronic lung disease
- cardiac transplantation.

1. Is the RV dilated?

- This may be a new finding. Significant RV dilatation is present if the RV is as large as or larger than the normal LV in the apical 4-chamber view.
- A simple set of thresholds is given in Table 10.1 (and see Figure 10.1) and more detailed measurements in Appendix 1.

Table 10.1 Thresholds for abnormal RV size in diastole[1,2]

	Dilated[a]
Tricuspid annulus (cm)	>3.0
Maximum transverse (cm)	>4.0
Base-to-apex (cm)	>9.0

[a]These values are derived from two sets of normal ranges

2. If large, is the RV active or hypokinetic?

- An active RV suggests an ASD shunt or tricuspid or pulmonary regurgitation (Table 10.2).
- A hypokinetic RV suggests pulmonary hypertension, myocardial infarction, or a myopathy or long-standing severe pulmonary or tricuspid regurgitation (Table 10.2).
- Look for a regional abnormality of contraction, and also check the inferior wall of the LV, since about a third of inferior LV infarcts are associated with RV infarction.

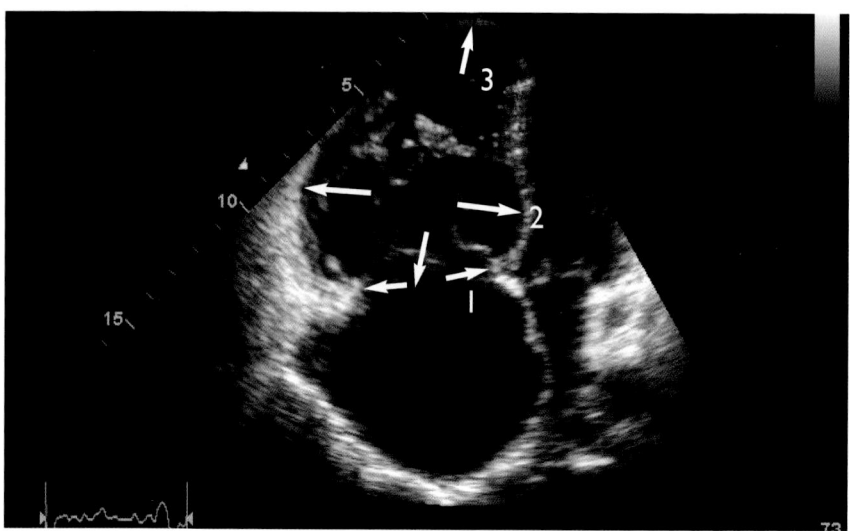

Figure 10.1 Levels for measuring RV size. 1 is at the annulus, 2 is the maximum transverse diameter, and 3 is base-to-apex. This is a 4-chamber view centred on the RV in a patient with arrhythmogenic RV dysplasia

Table 10.2 Causes of RV dilatation

Active
- Left-to-right shunt above the RV
- Tricuspid or pulmonary regurgitation

Hypokinetic
- Pulmonary hypertension, especially acute pulmonary embolism
- RV infarction
- RV myopathy
- End-stage pulmonary valve disease or tricuspid regurgitation

3. Quantification of systolic function using long-axis measurements

- Place the M-mode cursor on the junction between the RV free wall and tricuspid annulus in a 4-chamber view. Measure the excursion as the vertical distance between the peak and nadir (tricuspid annular plane systolic excursion: TAPSE) (Figure 10.2 and Table 10.3).
- Place the Doppler tissue sample in the RV free wall at the tricuspid annulus (Figure 10.3 and Table 10.3). Record the peak systolic velocity. A velocity <11.6 cm/s suggests a reduced RV ejection fraction or pulmonary hypertension.[3,4]

Table 10.3 Measures of RV function

Long-axis excursion (TAPSE)	
Normal range[5]	24.9 ± 3.5 mm
RV ejection fraction[6]	3.2 × long-axis excursion (mm)
Abnormal threshold[5]	<18 mm
Doppler tissue S velocity	
Normal range[3]	14.0 ± 2.8 cm/s
Normal range[4]	15.5 ± 2.6 cm/s
Abnormal threshold[3,4]	<11.6 cm/s

4. Is there RV hypertrophy?

This is defined by a free wall thickness >5 mm. RV hypertrophy suggests:

- Eisenmenger syndrome (pulmonary hypertension as a result of left-to-right shunting)
- pulmonary stenosis
- hypertrophic cardiomyopathy
- amyloid.

5. Is there left-sided disease?

- RV dilatation as a result of pulmonary hypertension may complicate severe mitral stenosis, but can also occur in end-stage aortic stenosis and occasionally mitral regurgitation.

92 Echocardiography: A Practical Guide for Reporting

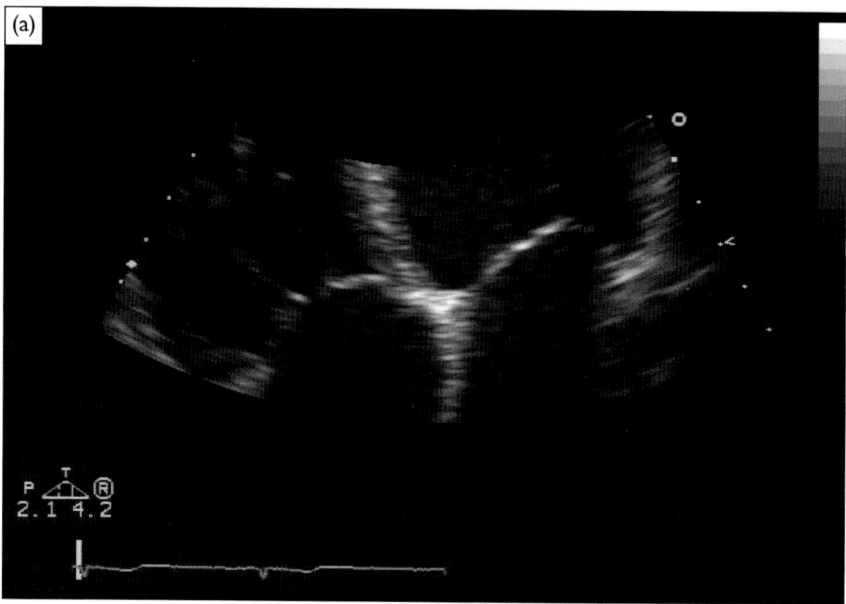

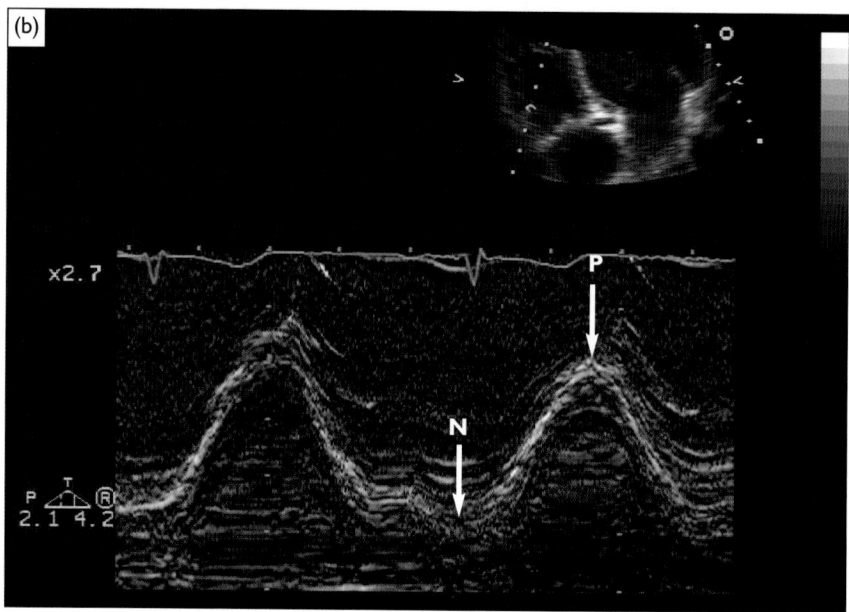

Figure 10.2 Long-axis excursion. Position for placing the M-mode cursor and the M-mode recording obtained. Measure from nadir (N) to peak (P)

Right heart 93

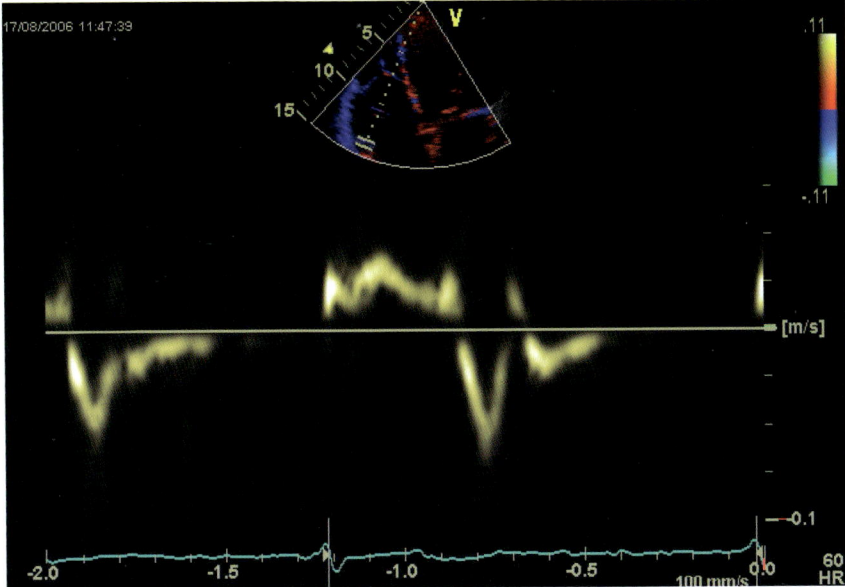

Figure 10.3 Doppler tissue imaging. Position for placing the cursor and the recording obtained

6. Is there evidence of a shunt above the RV?

- If the RV is dilated and active, but no ASD is visible, injection of agitated saline may show an ASD as a void caused by a left-to-right jet or by the right-to-left passage of microcavitation.
- Otherwise consider TOE, which is usually necessary to detect a sinus venosus defect or partial anomalous pulmonary venous drainage.

7. Is there tricuspid and pulmonary regurgitation?

See pages 59 and 61.

Checklist for reporting the RV

1. RV size and systolic function
2. Pulmonary pressures
3. Right-sided valve disease
4. Evidence of a shunt
5. Presence of left-sided disease

8. Estimate pulmonary artery pressure
See below.

PULMONARY HYPERTENSION

1. Estimating systolic pressure

- Measure the tricuspid regurgitant peak velocity V_{max}. If the signal varies, take the highest value. Estimate the pressure difference ($4V_{max}^2$).
- Estimate the RA pressure range from the response of the IVC (subcostal view) to inspiration (Table 10.4).
- The sum of these two is the RV systolic pressure. This is the same as the pulmonary systolic pressure, assuming that there is no pulmonary stenosis.

Table 10.4 Semisubjective estimation of RA pressure from the IVC

Collapse on inspiration	Pressure estimate (mmHg)
Complete	0–5
>50%	5–10
25–50%	10–15
<25%	15–20

- With severe tricuspid regurgitation, pressures >20 mmHg may often occur
- IVC diameter is probably too variable to be a firm guide

2. Estimating diastolic pressure

- Measure the end-diastolic velocity of the pulmonary regurgitant signal V_{ED} (Figure 10.4) and estimate the pressure difference ($4V_{ED}^2$).
- Estimate the RA pressure (Table 10.4).
- The sum of these is the pulmonary artery diastolic pressure (assuming no tricuspid stenosis).

3. Detection of pulmonary hypertension if there is no measurable tricuspid regurgitant jet

- Place the pulsed sample in the centre of the main PA or the pulmonary valve annulus. Avoid placing the sample too near the artery wall, which may give an artefactually sharp signal.

Right heart

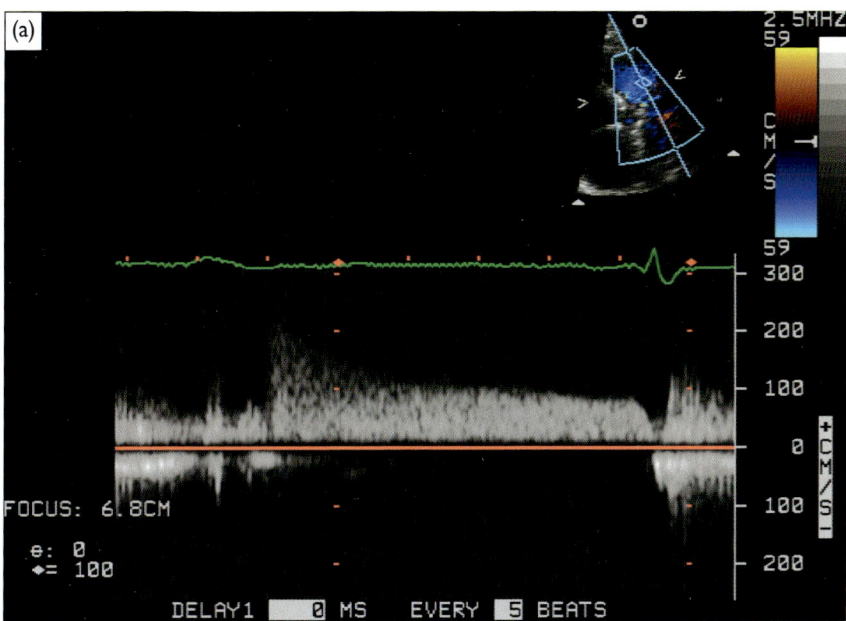

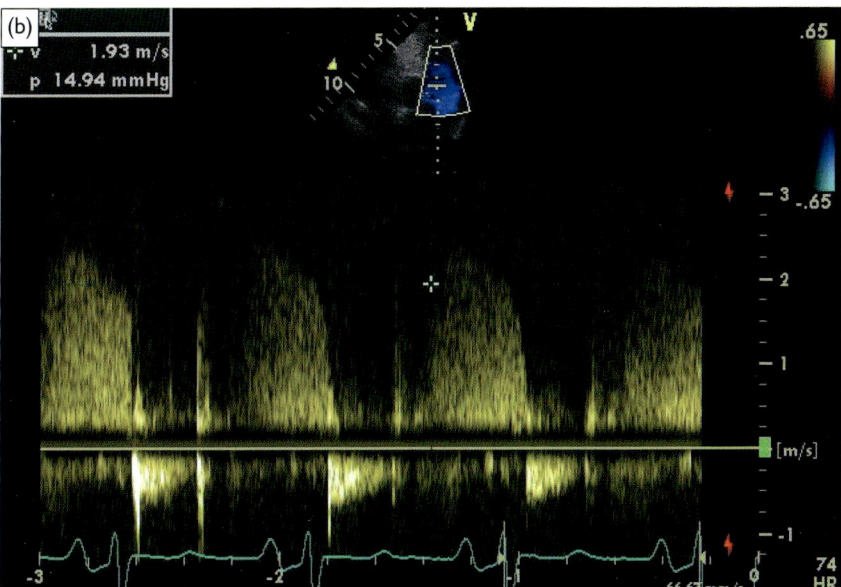

Figure 10.4 Pulmonary regurgitation. PA diastolic pressure is estimated using the end-diastolic velocity of the pulmonary regurgitant continuous-wave signal added to an estimate of RA pressure. (a) was recorded in a normal subject and (b) in a patient with pulmonary hypertension in whom the end-diastolic velocity was 2.0 mls

- Measure the time from the start of flow to the peak velocity (Figure 10.5).
- A time >105 ms excludes pulmonary hypertension[7] while a time <80 ms makes pulmonary hypertension highly likely. This method is not accurate enough to give an estimate of absolute pressure.

4. Estimating RV systolic pressure with a VSD

- Measure the brachial artery systolic pressure and subtract $4V_{VSD}^2$, where V_{VSD} is the peak velocity across the VSD.

5. Assess RV size and systolic function

See page 89.

6. Assess grade of tricuspid regurgitation

See page 59.

7. Look for cardiac causes of pulmonary hypertension (Table 10.5)

- Some of the extracardiac causes may also affect the echocardiogram (Table 10.5).

Table 10.5 Causes of pulmonary hypertension

Cardiac
- Left-sided disease:
  - Mitral valve disease
  - Severe aortic stenosis
  - Severe left ventricular impairment
- Congenital heart disease

Extracardiac
- Thromboembolic disease
- Chronic lung disease
- Autoimmune disease e.g. SLE (also associated with valve thickening, LV dilatation, pericardial effusion)
- Scleroderma
- HIV (also causes LV dilatation)
- Drugs, e.g. anorexic agents (also cause valve thickening)
- Primary pulmonary hypertension

Right heart

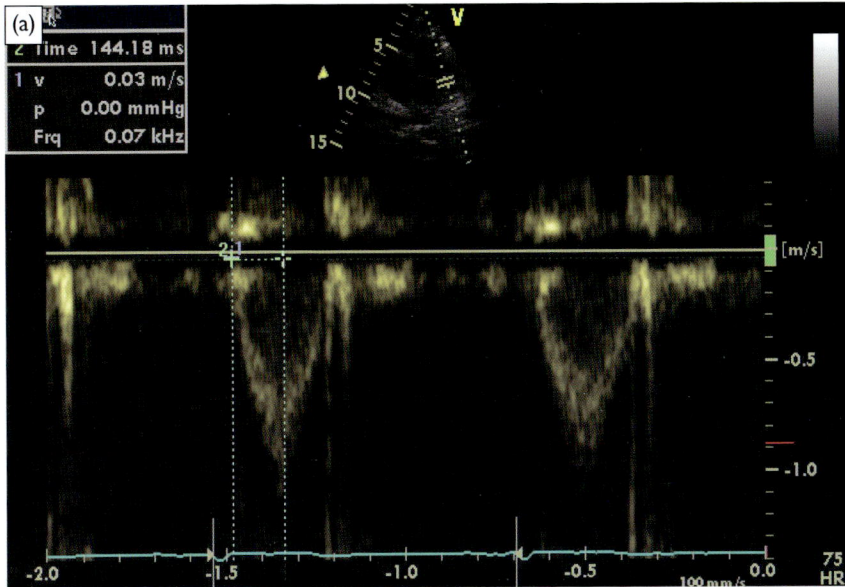

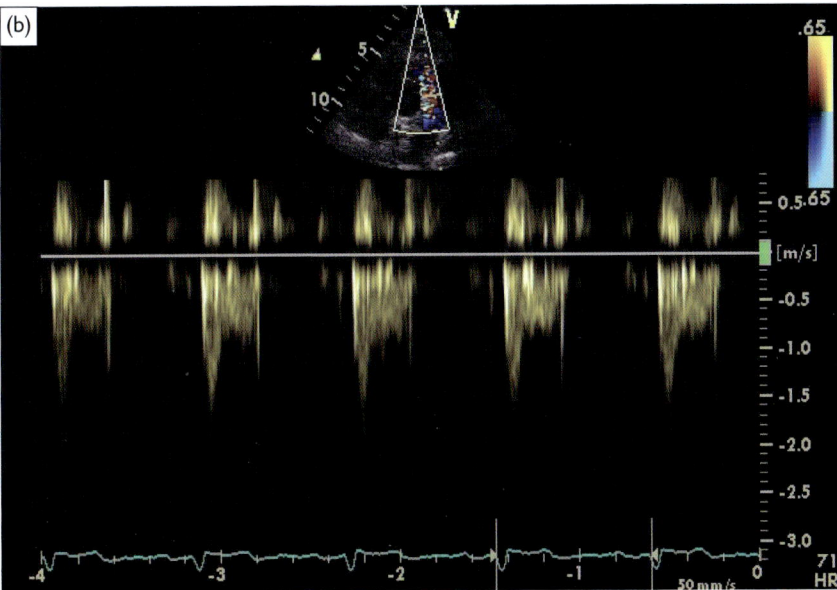

Figure 10.5 PA velocity. A normal waveform with time to peak velocity 144 ms (a) and a recording in a patient with pulmonary hypertension (b). The time to peak velocity is short and the signal is notched as a result of increased wave reflectance

> **Checklist for reporting pulmonary hypertension**
>
> 1. Estimated pulmonary pressures or presence/absence based on time to peak PA velocity
> 2. RV size and systolic function
> 3. Tricuspid regurgitation grade
> 4. Underlying cause?

REFERENCES

1. Triulzi MO, Gillam LD, Gentile F. Normal adult cross-sectional echocardiographic values: linear dimensions and chamber areas. Echocardiography 1984; 1:403–26.
2. Foale R, Nihoyannopoulos P, McKenna W, et al. Echocardiographic measurement of the normal adult right ventricle. Br Heart J 1986; 56:33–44.
3. Gin PL, Wang WC, Yang SH, Hsiao SH, Tseng JC. Right heart function in systemic lupus erythematosus: insights from myocardial Doppler tissue imaging. J Am Soc Echocardiogr 2006; 19:441–9.
4. Meluzin J, Spinarova L, Bakala J, et al. Pulsed Doppler tissue imaging of the velocity of tricuspid annular systolic motion; a new, rapid, and non-invasive method of evaluating right ventricular systolic function. Eur Heart J 2001; 22:340–8.
5. Hammarstrom E, Wranne B, Pinto FJ, Purvear J, Popp RL. Tricuspid annular motion. J Am Soc Echo 1991; 4:131–9.
6. Kaul S, Tei C, Hopkins JM, Shah PM. Assessment of right ventricular function using two-dimensional echocardiography. Am Heart J 1984; 107:526–31.
7. Kosturakis D, Goldberg SJ, Allen HD, Loeber C. Doppler echocardiographic prediction of pulmonary arterial hypertension in congenital heart disease. Am J Cardiol 1984; 53:1110–15.

11 ADULT CONGENITAL DISEASE

SIMPLE DEFECTS

1. ASD

- The diagnosis should be considered if the RV is dilated.
- Describe the position. Most are approximately in the centre of the septum (secundum). 'Primum' defects (correctly termed partial AV septal defects) are next to the AV valves (Table 11.1).
- It is possible to mistake flow from the SVC for flow across an ASD. Take multiple views. If there is still doubt, consider a contrast injection or TOE or use pulsed Doppler on the RA side of the septum. ASD flow has a peak in late diastole and systole. For the SVC, the peaks are earlier.
- Calculate the shunt as the ratio of flow in the PA to the LV outflow tract (Table 11.2).
- Estimate the PA pressure (page 94).
- TOE is indicated before device closure of a secundum ASD (Table 11.3) and TTE afterwards (Table 11.5).

Table 11.1 Features of a partial AV septal defect ('primum')

- Defect adjacent to the AV valves
- Common AV valve rather than separate tricuspid and mitral valves:
  - Lack of offset between left- and right-sided AV valve
  - Left AV valve appears 'cleft' or trileaflet
- Long LV outflow tract caused by an offset between aortic valve and 'mitral valve' (normally the non-coronary aortic cusp is continuous with the base of the anterior mitral leaflet)
- May be associated with a VSD

Table 11.2 Levels for shunt calculation[a]

	Downstream	Upstream
ASD	PA	LV outflow
VSD	PA	LV outflow
PDA	LV outflow	Pulmonary valve

[a] See page 138.

2. VSD

- Localise the site of the defect (Figure 11.1).
- Estimate the shunt (Table 11.2).
- Assess the LV. LV volume load suggests a large shunt. Volume overload and systolic dilatation are criteria for closure.
- Estimate PA pressures (page 94).

3. PDA

- Look for reversed flow in the main PA using parasternal short- and long-axis views and for the defect in the suprasternal view (Figure 11.2a).
- Estimate the PA pressure (page 94). When this is raised, flow through the duct may diminish, cease, or reverse during systole. When it is normal, flow is continuous throughout the cardiac cycle (Figure 11.2b).
- Estimate the shunt size (Table 11.2). LV volume load suggests a large shunt.

4. Coarctation

See page 83.

SYSTEMATIC STUDY

- Congenital disease should be suspected if specific abnormalities are found (Table 11.4).
- Little or no background information may be available (e.g., new diagnosis, emergency admission, details of corrective surgery not available).

Adult congenital disease

Table 11.3 What to look for on TOE before device closure

- How many defects or fenestrations?
- Total septal length
- Diameter of defect on imaging and colour in 4-chamber and bicaval views
- Distance from AV valves
- Distance from IVC and SVC
- Distance from aorta (a margin is not necessary when an Amplatzer device is used)
- Check correct drainage or right-sided pulmonary veins
- Other cardiac abnormalities, e.g. mitral prolapse

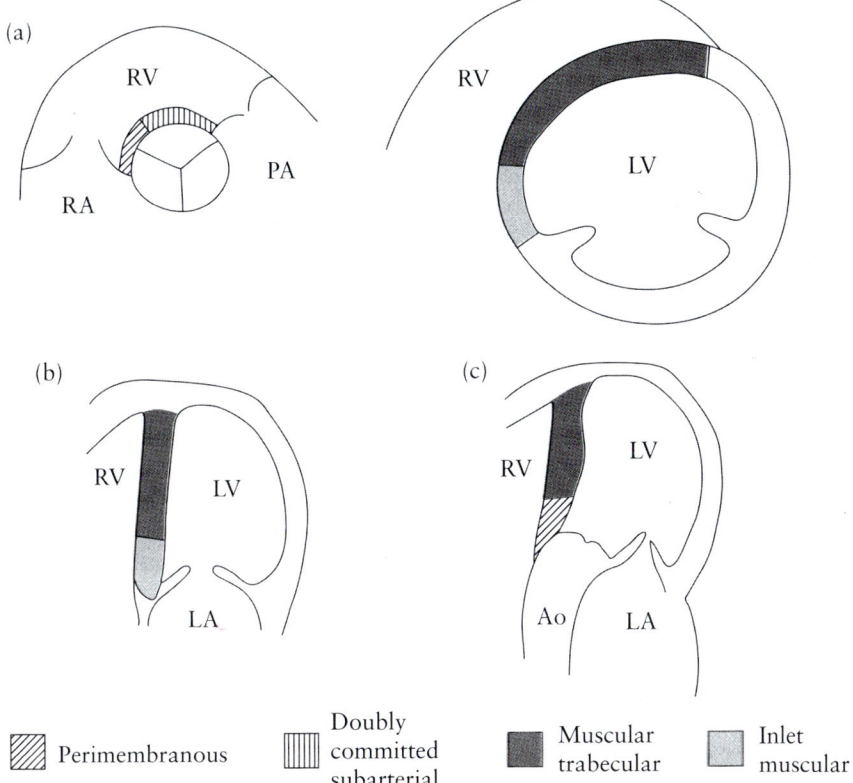

Figure 11.1 Position of VSDs. (a) Parasternal short-axis at aortic level. (b) Parasternal short-axis at papillary muscle level. (c) Apical 4-chamber. (d) Apical 5-chamber

Table 11.4 Findings suspicious of congenital disease

- Dilated or hypertrophied RV
- Pulmonary hypertension
- PA and aorta seen in cross-section in the same plane
- Hyperdynamic LV without aortic or mitral regurgitation
- Lack of off-setting between left and right AV valves (Figure 11.3)
- Dilated coronary sinus (Figure 11.4)

- Perform a systematic study, allowing a specialist review if necessary.
- 'AV valve' refers to the tricuspid and mitral valves and 'semilunar valve' to the pulmonary and aortic valves. Thus, 'left AV valve' makes no assumption that this is truly the mitral valve.
- 'Anatomic LV' means the ventricle on the left of the heart; 'morphologic LV' means the ventricle attached to the mitral valve.
- Discordant means incorrect connections – for example, LA attached to morphologic RV or aorta leading from morphologic RV.

1. Are the atria correctly positioned?

- The morphologic LA and RA are distinguished by their appendages. Since these may not be seen transthoracically, the relationship of the abdominal vessels ('situs') is used.
- Are the IVC and abdominal aorta normally related in an abdominal short-axis view?
- Follow the IVC (and SVC if visible) to the RA using subcostal views and check that this is on the correct side of the heart.

2. Are the atria attached to the correct ventricles?

- This is usually appreciated best from the apical 4-chamber view.
- The morphologic RV is recognised because:
  - its AV valve is more apical than the left-sided AV valve and it has a septal attachment
  - there is an offset between the AV valve and the semilunar valve
  - there are more trabeculations than in the morphologic LV
  - there is usually a moderator band.

3. Are the ventricles attached to the correct great arteries?

- The PA bifurcates early and the aorta has an arch giving off the head and neck branch arteries.

Adult congenital disease 103

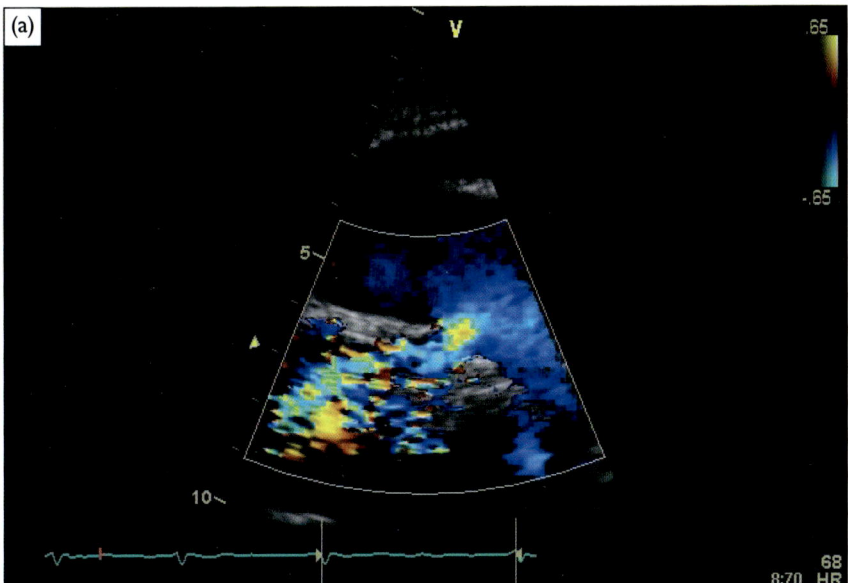

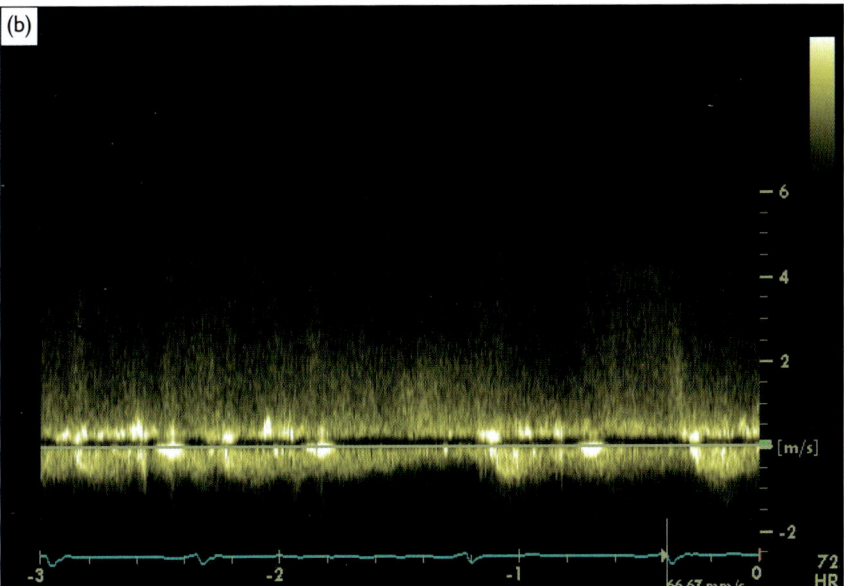

Figure 11.2 PDA. The defect from a suprasternal position (a) and on continuous-wave (b) from a parasternal window in a large duct with normal pulmonary pressures

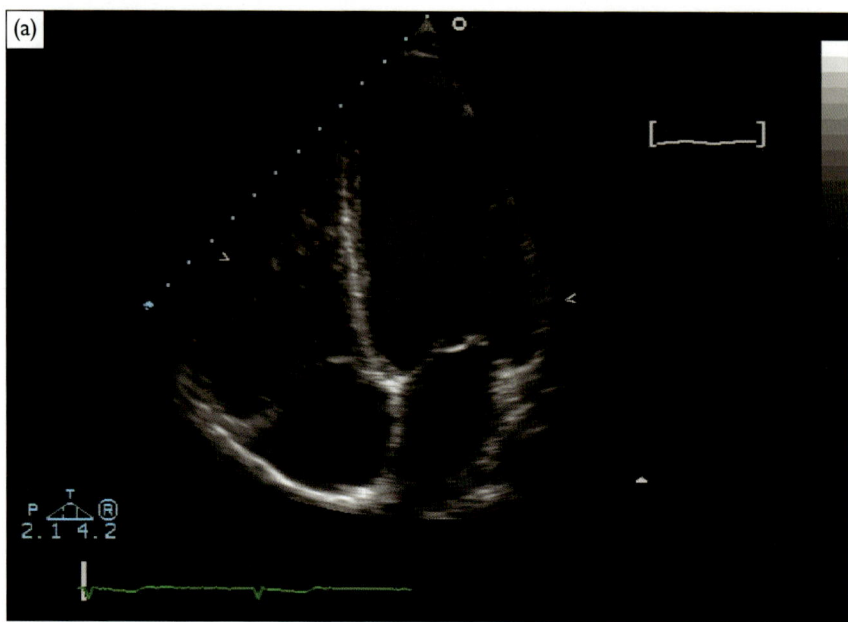

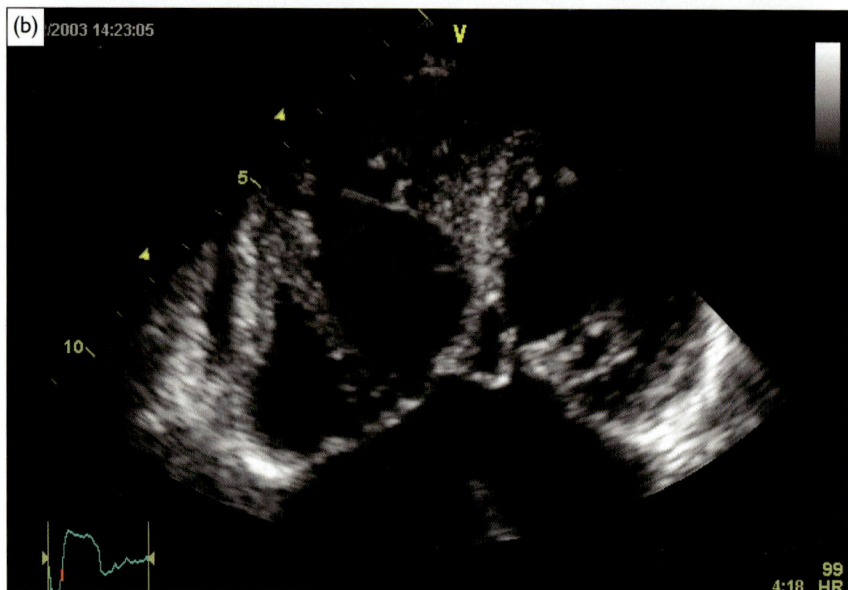

Figure 11.3 AVSD. (a) A normal 4-chamber view showing that the tricuspid valve is offset or closer to the apex than the mitral valve. (b) Here there is lack of offsetting, implying that there is a common AV valve. In addition, there is a large ASD.

- Congenitally corrected transposition of the great arteries is suspected if both great vessels can be imaged in transverse section from a parasternal short-axis view or longitudinally in a subcostal view.

4. Assess the size and systolic function of both ventricles
(pages 5 and 89)

- It is usual for a morphologic RV connected to the systemic circulation to be dilated.

5. Estimate PA pressure (page 94)

- Make sure to assess the AV valve jet from the ventricle connected to the pulmonary circulation.
- If there is outflow obstruction from valve stenosis or a band, the calculated pressures will reflect RV and not PA systolic pressure.

6. Are there any shunts at atrial or ventricular level?

- Measure size anatomically and estimate the shunt (page 138).

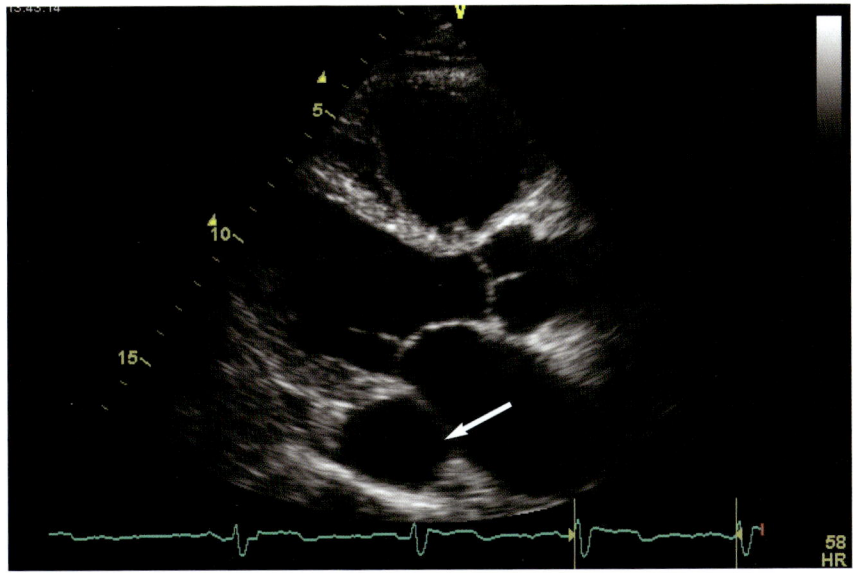

Figure 11.4 Dilated coronary sinus (arrow). This is usually caused by a left-sided SVC

7. Are the cardiac valves normal in appearance?

- Assess stenosis and regurgitation as for acquired valve disease.
- If there is no offsetting of the AV valves, the diagnosis is likely to be an AVSD (Figure 11.3).

8. Is there aortic coarctation or a PDA?

See pages 83 and 100.

9. Are the origins of the coronary arteries correctly positioned?

Table 11.5 TTE after device-closure of an ASD or PFO

- Position of device
- Is there any residual atrial shunt? A small central leak through the device is normal and will disappear with time.
- Does the device obstruct the IVC or SVC?
- Is the device close to the mitral valve and is there new or worse mitral regurgitation?
- RV size and function (size may start to fall soon after closure)
- Pericardial effusion (as a sign of perforation during the procedure)

Table 11.6 Transthoracic study after closure of a VSD or PDA

- Is there a residual shunt? If more than trivial, perform a shunt calculation
- LV size and function
- Aortic regurgitation if closure of perimembranous VSD
- PA pressure

Table 11.7 Transthoracic study after coarctation repair or stenting

- Is there a residual, new or in-stent stenosis on imaging?
- On continuous-wave, an elevated systolic velocity is normal, but there should be no diastolic forward flow
- Assess the aorta beyond the repair, looking for aneurysmal dilatation
- Assess the ascending aorta and aortic valve if bicuspid

10. Is the coronary sinus dilated? (Figure 11.4)

- This is usually caused by a left-sided SVC (image from the medial edge of the left supraclavicular fossa), occasionally by insertion of an aberrant coronary artery.

POST-PROCEDURE STUDIES

- Checklists are given for the echocardiogram after:
  - device-closure of an ASD or PFO (Table 11.5)
  - closure of VSD or PDA (Table 11.6)
  - coarctation repair (Table 11.7)
  - Fallot repair (Table 11.8)
  - Mustard–Senning procedures (Table 11.9)
- If the procedure is unknown, then perform a systematic examination (page 100).

Table 11.8 Transthoracic study after repair of tetralogy of Fallot[a]

- Situs
- RV size and function, including RV pressure
- Is the VSD patch fully competent?
- Aortic dimensions (looking for aortic dilatation)
- Assess pulmonary valve for stenosis and regurgitation
- Assess branch PA flow on colour and pulsed Doppler if possible
- Assess the RV outflow tract for muscular hypertrophy

[a]Over-riding aorta with VSD, RV outflow obstruction, with RV hypertrophy

Table 11.9 Mustard–Senning procedures[a]

- Check unobstructed flow (V_{max} <1.5 m/s) through the IVC and SVC arms of the baffle to mitral valve, then LV, then PA (Figure 11.5a)
- Check unobstructed flow of pulmonary venous return (V_{max} <1.5 m/s) to the tricuspid valve, then RV, then aorta (Figure 11.5b)
- Check for baffle leak
- LV size and function (expected to be small)
- Systemic RV size and function (expected to be dilated)

[a]For transposition of the great arteries

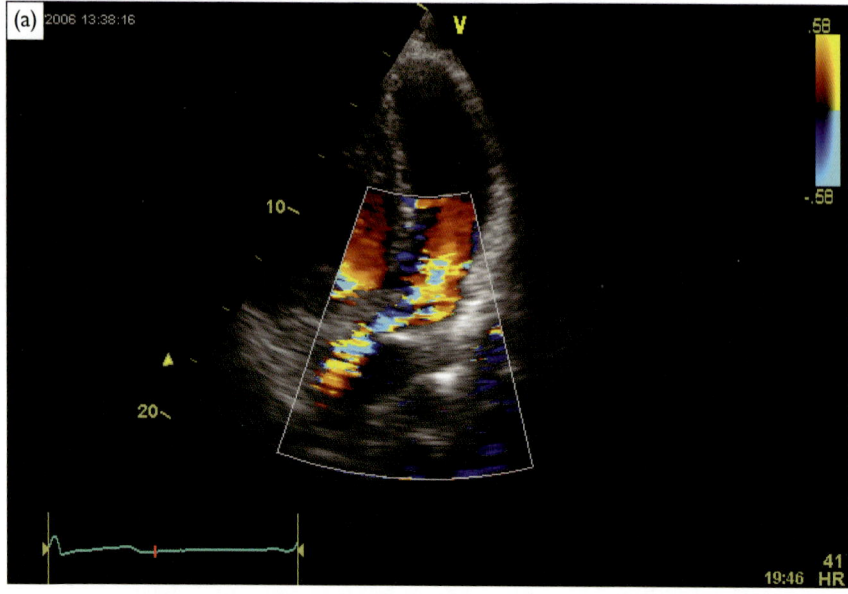

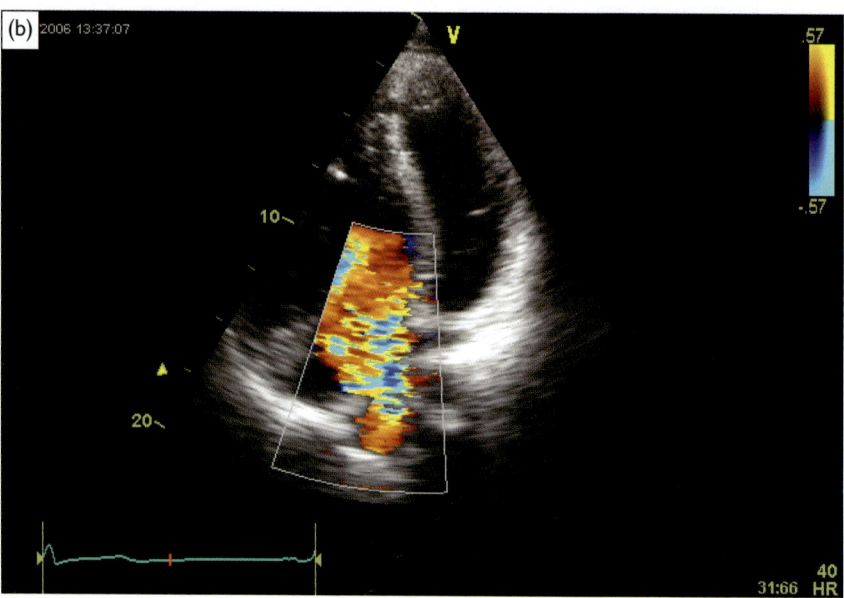

Figure 11.5 Appearance after the Mustard procedure. There is unobstructed flow from the great veins to the mitral valve (a) and from the pulmonary veins to the RV (b)

12 PERICARDIAL EFFUSION

1. Pericardial or pleural?

See Table 12.1 and Figure 12.1.

Table 12.1 Differential diagnosis of pericardial and pleural effusions

Pericardial	Pleural
Ends anterior to the descending aorta	Ends posterior to the descending aorta
Minor overlapping of LA	May significantly overlap LA
Fluid between heart and diaphragm on subcostal view	No fluid between heart and diaphragm on subcostal view
Tamponade may be present	No signs of tamponade
Rarely >4 cm	May be >4 cm
If large, swinging of the heart	Heart fixed

2. Size and distribution

- *Size (Table 12.2) is far less important than whether there are signs of tamponade (Table 12.3).*

Table 12.2 Guideline to effusion size by maximum separation of the pericardial layers

Small	Moderate	Large
<1 cm	1–3 cm	>3 cm

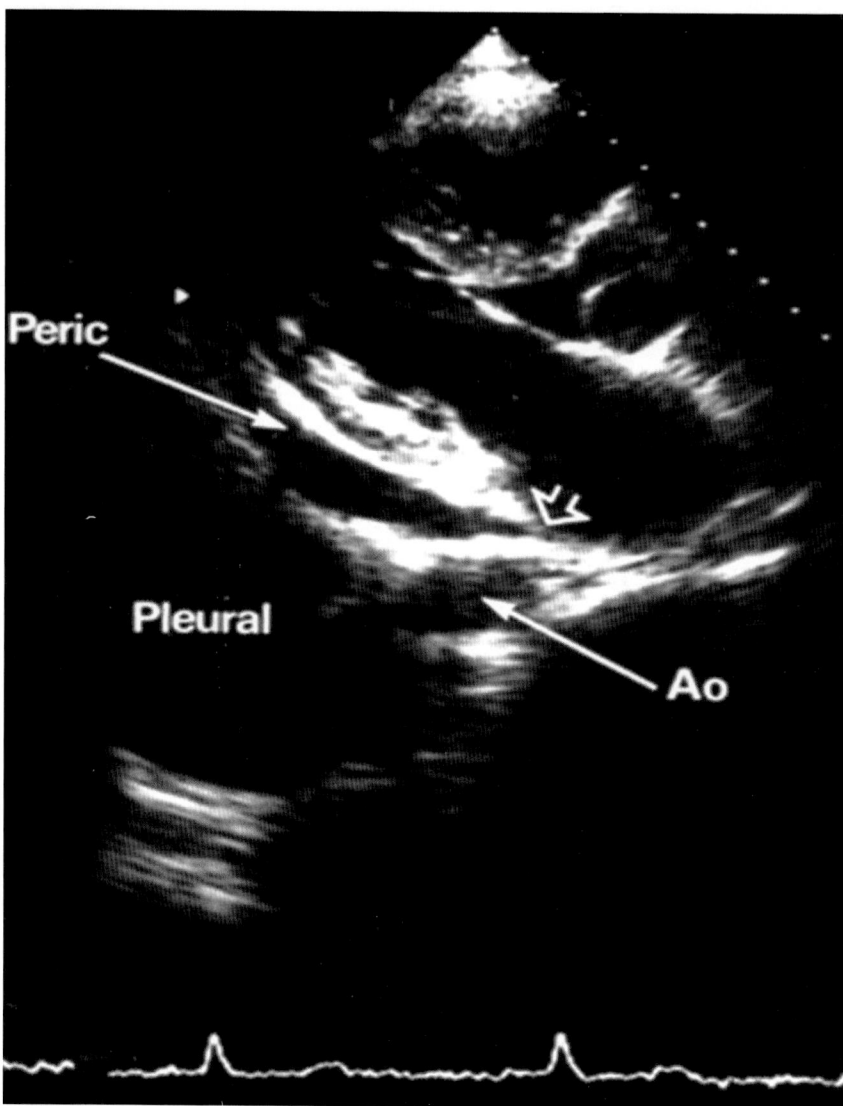

Figure 12.1 Pericardial versus pleural fluid. A pericardial effusion ends anterior to the descending thoracic aorta (arrow); a pleural effusion ends posterior to the aorta. A pleural effusion may extend over the LA; a pericardial effusion never does to any significant degree

Pericardial effusion

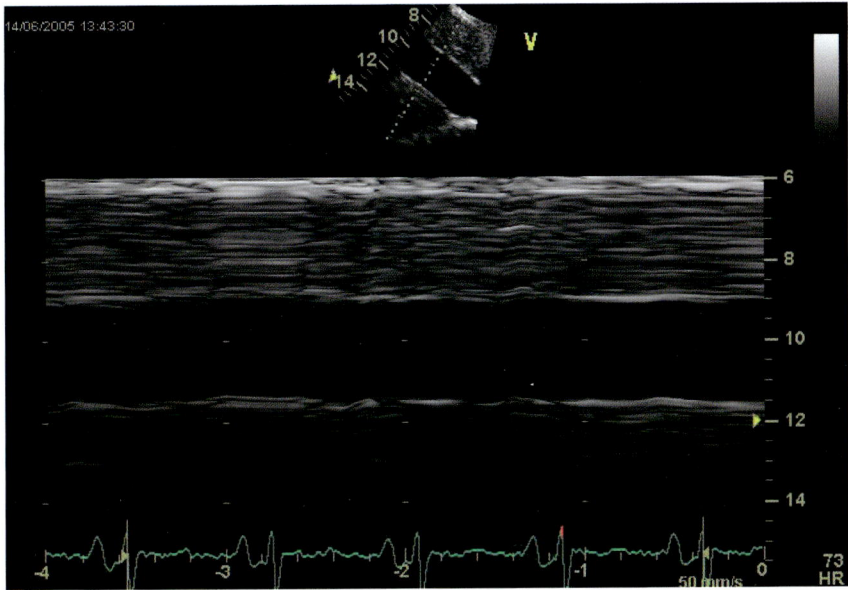

Figure 12.2 Engorged inferior vena cava. There is little change in diameter throughout the respiratory cycle or after a sniff

Table 12.3 Echocardiographic evidence of tamponade

- Dilated IVC (>2 cm) with inspiratory collapse of <50% (Figure 12.2)
- Fall in aortic or early diastolic mitral velocity during inspiration >25% (Figure 12.3)[1]
- Prolonged and widespread diastolic RV collapse
- Note that collapse of the RA and RV outflow tract are non-specific signs

- Is the effusion generalised/posterior/apical/anterior?
- *Is there enough fluid in the subcostal view for safe pericardiocentesis (usually >2 cm)?*
- What is the consistency of the fluid? Echodense collections may not drain via a needle. Localised strands and masses are common if the protein content is high, and do not usually represent a separate pathology (e.g. metastasis).

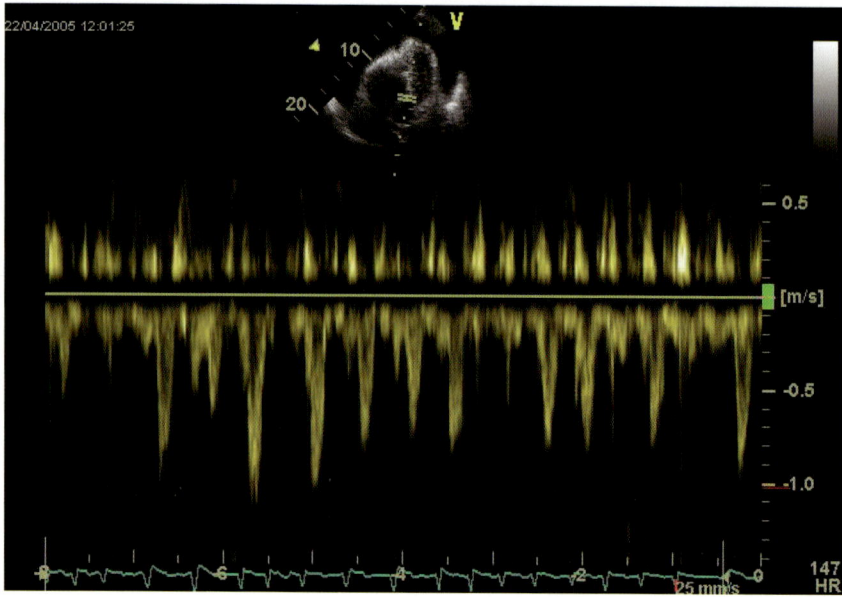

Figure 12.3 Increased paradox. The subaortic peak velocity falls by >25% during inspiration.

3. Is tamponade present?

See Table 12.3.

4. General

- Is LV function poor? (Pericardiocentesis may cause circulatory collapse.)
- If the effusion is small but there is respiratory variability of left-sided velocities or the patient is significantly breathless, consider effusive–constrictive pericarditis (a mixture of effusion and pericardial constriction).
- If the pericardial region looks abnormal but there is no obvious effusion, consider the causes listed in Table 12.4.
- In patients with unexplained hypotension after cardiac surgery, look for localised effusion or haematoma, e.g. over the atria (usually requires TOE).

Table 12.4 Causes of an abnormal pericardial region

- Pericardial cyst
- Haematoma – usually after surgery or trauma
- Fat – this causes a layer of moderate echogenicity, usually anteriorly and usually in obese subjects
- LV pseudo-aneurysm (page 25)
- Extrinsic mass
- Oesophageal hernia

Checklist for reporting pericardial effusion
1. Size and distribution
2. Evidence of tamponade
3. Is there enough fluid in the direction of proposed drainage
4. LV function

REFERENCE

1. Goldstein JA. Cardiac tamponade, constrictive pericarditis, and restrictive cardiomyopathy. Curr Prob Cardiol 2004; 29:503–67.

13 MASSES

1. Describe the characteristics of the mass

See Table 13.1.

Table 13.1 Characteristics of the mass

- Site and attachment
- Size, shape
- Density (low intensity, dense, mixed)
- Mobility (fixed, mobile, free)

2. A mass attached to a valve

- This can be globular or thin (Table 13.2).

Table 13.2 Mass attached to a valve

Globular
- Vegetation
- Fibroelastoma
- Myxomatous tissue

Thin
- Ruptured chord
- Fibrin strand

3. LA or RA mass

- A mass attached to the atrial septum is likely to be a myxoma.
- A fixed mass attached away from the septum is likely to be malignant. An associated pericardial effusion makes an angiosarcoma likely.
- For an RA mass, check the IVC for tumour extension from a primary in the kidney or ovaries. Thrombus from a DVT may also appear in the IVC. Typically, a tumour will cause IVC dilatation, while a thrombus will not.
- For a sessile LA mass, check the pulmonary veins and look for a tumour mass outside the heart.
- LA thrombus is unlikely without a substrate (dilated LA, mitral stenosis).
- For causes of a non-pathologic atrial structure, see Table 13.3.

Table 13.3 Non-pathologic RA 'masses'

- Chiari membrane or net
- Eustachian valve
- Atrial septal aneurysm
- Atrial septal fat
- Pacemaker electrode
- Long central line

4. LV or RV mass (Table 13.4)

Table 13.4 Causes of LV or RV masses

- Thrombus
- Endomyocardial fibrosis
- Metastasis
- Primary tumour (e.g. rhabdomyosarcoma)
- Sarcoid

- Characteristics of thrombus are given on page 24. If there is uncertainty, use different views and consider transpulmonary contrast.
- Could the mass be normal? (Table 13.5)

Table 13.5 Normal LV or RV 'masses'

- Trabeculation
- Prominent RV moderator band
- LV false tendon
- Prominent papillary muscle

5. Extrinsic masses

See Table 13.6.

Table 13.6 Masses outside the heart

- Tumour
- Hiatus hernia
- Lymph node
- Haematoma
- Pericardial cyst
- Subdiaphragmatic masses (e.g. polycystic kidney)

6. Haemodynamic effect

- Assess the presence and degree of valve regurgitation or obstruction to inflow, depending on the site of the mass.

Checklist for reporting a mass
1. Location and site of attachment
2. Size and density
3. Mobility
4. Involvement of adjacent veins
5. Haemodynamic effect

14 GENERAL

SPECIFIC CLINICAL REQUESTS

The request form may not specify what to look for on the echocardiogram, and this chapter provides lists for a focused study or part of a standard study.

Emergency echocardiography

This may be requested for the following:

- cardiac arrest (Table 14.1)
- collapse with suspected pulmonary embolism (Table 14.2)
- hypotension after an invasive cardiac procedure (including central line insertion): look for the following:

Table 14.1 Focused list for echocardiography after cardiac arrest

- LV function:
  - Global dysfunction
  - Regional wall motion abnormality
  - Hypertrophy
- Acute complications of infarction:
  - Flail mitral valve
  - Ventricular septal rupture
  - Free wall rupture
- RV dilatation (see Table 14.2)
- Pericardial tamponade
- Severe aortic stenosis
- Obstructed prosthetic valve
- Aortic dissection rupturing into pleural space or abdominal cavity

Table 14.2 Echocardiographic signs of massive pulmonary embolism[1]

- RV dilatation and free wall hypokinesis
- Tricuspid regurgitation V_{max} usually <4.0 m/s
- Short time to PA V_{max} <60 ms
- IVC dilated and unreactive
- Occasionally thrombus in the PA or right heart

- pericardial effusion
- signs of tamponade (may be present even if the effusion is small)
- other causes of hypotension (Table 14.3).

Urgent echocardiography

This may be requested for the following:
- trauma (Table 14.4)
- hypotension (Table 14.3)
- hypotension after cardiac surgery (Table 14.5)
- hypoxaemia:
  - causes of hypotension (Table 14.3)
  - contrast study for right-to-left shunting at atrial level.

Table 14.3 Focused list in hypotension

Signs of underfilling
- Flat IVC
- Small and active RV and LV
- Low E and A wave on transmitral pulsed Doppler

Cardiogenic causes
- LV global or regional dysfunction
- RV dysfunction (see also Table 14.2)
- Pericardial tamponade
- Severe valve lesions

Sepsis
- LV dilated and hypokinetic
- RV dilated and hypokinetic

Table 14.4 Focused list for echocardiography after blunt or penetrating trauma

Blunt
- Pericardial effusion
- Contusion
  - RV dilatation and hypokinesis
  - Localised LV thickening and wall motion abnormality, especially anteroapically
- Ventricular septal rupture
- Regional wall motion abnormality (dissected coronary artery)
- Valve rupture causing acute mitral or tricuspid regurgitation, occasionally aortic regurgitation
- Aortic dilatation and dissection flap or intramural haematoma (TOE)
- Aortic transection (TOE)

Penetrating
- RV wall hypokinesis
- VSD
- Pericardial effusion or haematoma (which may be localised)
- Pleural fluid
- Mitral regurgitation from valve laceration or damage to papillary muscle or chordae
- Aortic regurgitation from laceration of aortic valve

Table 14.5 Focused list for echocardiography in hypotension after cardiac surgery

- LV global and regional systolic function
- Hypertrophic cardiomyopathy-like physiology after aortic valve replacement for aortic stenosis with small LV cavity and LV outflow acceleration
- RV size and systolic function
- Prosthetic valve regurgitation or obstruction
- Native valve function
- Pericardial tamponade
- Localised haematoma over atria (TOE)
- Signs of underfilling (Table 14.3)

Table 14.6 Ventricular tachycardia

- LV systolic and diastolic function
- Localised abnormalities (e.g. metastases)
- LV hypertrophy?
- RV dysplasia (see page 35)

Table 14.7 Atrial fibrillation

- LA and RA size
- LA thrombus?
- LV size and function
- Mitral valve appearance and function
- RV size and function
- PA pressures
- Mitral valve appearance and function

Table 14.8 Heart failure

- LV cavity size and wall thickness
- LV systolic and diastolic function
- RV function and PA pressure
- IVC size and response to respiration
- Valve appearance and function

Table 14.9 Stroke, TIA, or peripheral embolism

- LV size and systolic function
- Signs of hypertension
  - LV hypertrophy
  - LV diastolic dysfunction
  - Dilated LA
  - Dilated aorta
- Mitral valve disease
- PFO
- Intracardiac masses

Other focused lists

See Tables 14.6–14.15.

Table 14.10 Cocaine

Acute
- Wall motion abnormality (myocardial infarction)
- Generalised LV hypokinesis (myocarditis)
- Aortic dissection

Long-term use
- Dilated LV
- LV hypertrophy
- Evidence of endocarditis

Table 14.11 HIV

- Dilated LV
- Pulmonary hypertension
- Pericardial effusion
- Evidence of endocarditis
- Pericardial thickening (e.g. Kaposi sarcoma, non-Hodgkin lymphoma)

Table 14.12 Murmur: ? cause

- Thickening or regurgitation of all four valves
- Subaortic membrane
- Hypertrophic cardiomyopathy
- RV outflow hypertrophy
- Coarctation
- PDA
- VSD
- ASD
- PA membrane (rare)

Table 14.13 Hypertension

- LV cavity size, wall thickness
- LV mass
- LV systolic and diastolic function
- LA size
- Aortic dimensions
- Aortic valve thickening

Table 14.14 Chronic renal failure

- LV hypertrophy
- LV dilatation and hypokinesis
- Dysplastic calcification:
  – Aortic valve thickening
  – Mitral annular calcification
  – Aortic calcification
- Pulmonary hypertension
- Pericardial effusion

Table 14.15 Systemic lupus erythematosus

- Valve thickening, including localised vegetations
- Calcified or ruptured chordae
- LV dysfunction (myocarditis, myocardial infarction)
- Pericardial effusion
- Atrial or ventricular masses

INDICATIONS FOR URGENT CLINICAL ADVICE

See Table 14.16.

Table 14.16 Examples of findings at echocardiography requiring urgent clinical advice

- Post-myocardial infarction complication:
  - VSD
  - Papillary muscle rupture
  - Pseudoaneurysm
- RV dilatation in a hypotensive patient (possible acute pulmonary embolism)
- Aortic dissection
- Pericardial effusion (especially if large or with associated tamponade):
- Critical valve disease
- Myxoma or ball thrombus
- LV thrombus
- Unexpected vegetation

INDICATIONS FOR FURTHER ECHOCARDIOGRAPHY

See Tables 14.17–14.19.

Table 14.17 Examples of indications for contrast echocardiography

Agitated saline or gelofusin
- PFO:
  - Stroke or TIA in a young subject
  - Diver
  - Migraine
- Improving incomplete tricuspid regurgitant signal for the estimation of PA pressure

Transpulmonary contrast
- Poor endocardial definition:
  - Stress echocardiography
  - Measurement of LV ejection fraction
  - Diagnosis of LV dysfunction
- Thrombus
- Apical hypertrophic cardiomyopathy

Table 14.18 Examples of indications for TOE

- Suspected endocarditis:
  - In most cases of prosthetic valve endocarditis
  - When the transthoracic study is non-diagnostic
- Cerebral infarction, TIA, peripheral embolism:
  - Patients aged <50 years
  - Patients aged >50 years without evidence of cerebrovascular disease or other obvious cause in whom the findings of echocardiography will change management (e.g. to start warfarin if a PFO is found)
- Before cardioversion:
  - Previous cardioembolic event
  - Anticoagulation contraindicated
  - Atrial fibrillation of <48 hours' duration in the presence of structural heart disease
- Prosthetic valve:
  - To improve quantification of mitral regurgitation
  - Obstruction: to determine the cause
  - Uncertain obstruction on transthoracic imaging
  - Suspected endocarditis
  - Abnormal regurgitation suspected but TTE normal or equivocal (breathless patient, hyperdynamic LV, haemolytic anaemia)
  - Recurrent thrombembolism despite adequate anticoagulation
- Native valve disease:
  - To determine feasibility and safety of balloon mitral valvotomy
  - To determine whether a regurgitant mitral valve is repairable
- ASD:
  - To determine whether percutaneous closure is possible
- Aorta:
  - To diagnose dissection, intramural haematoma, or transection
  - To determine the size of the aorta (if transthoracic imaging inadequate)
- Perioperative:
  - To confirm preoperative diagnosis (e.g. suitability of mitral valve for repair)
  - Emergency surgery needed with insufficient time for full preoperative assessment, e.g. myocardial ischaemia, complications of infarct, aortic dissection
  - Assess unexpected findings at surgery, e.g. aortic regurgitation
  - To detect myocardial ischaemia during cardiac or noncardiac surgery
  - To assess mitral valve or aortic valve repair
  - To assess myomectomy
  - Difficulty in weaning off bypass, arrhythmias, hypotension
  - To confirm de-airing after bypass
  - To assess the haemodynamically unstable patient on ITU

Table 14.19 Indications and contraindications for stress echocardiography[2,3]

- Prediction of coronary disease in patients unsuitable for exercise testing (e.g. resting ECG changes, unable to walk) or at low risk of coronary disease (e.g. women)
- Risk stratification in known coronary disease (e.g. after myocardial infarction)
- After coronary angiography to assess functional significance of an equivocal lesion
- To assess adequacy of revacularisation (e.g. before non-cardiac surgery)
- To determine the presence of viability in apparently infarcted myocardium
- To assess valve disease (e.g. aortic stenosis with impaired LV, moderate aortic stenosis and non-specific symptoms, moderate mitral regurgitation but severe breathlessness)

REFERENCE

1. Kasper W, Geibel A, Tiede N, et al. Distinguishing between acute and subacute massive pulmonary embolism by conventional and Doppler echocardiography. Br Heart J 1993; 70:352–6.
2. Senior R, Monaghan M, Becher H, Mayet J, Nihoyannopoulos P, British Society of Echocardiography. Stress echocardiography for the diagnosis and risk stratification of patients with suspected or known coronary artery disease: a critical appraisal. Supported by the British Society of Echocardiography. Heart 91(4):427–36, 2005.
3. Becher H, Chambers J, Fox K, et al. BSE procedure guidelines for the clinical application of stress echocardiography, recommendations for performance and interpretation of stress echocardiography: a report for the British Society of Echocardiography Policy Committee. Heart 90(6):23–30, 2004.

APPENDICES

1. NORMAL RANGES FOR CARDIAC DIMENSIONS (Figure A1.1)

M-Mode:

1: LA
2: Aorta
3: IVS in diastole
4: PW in diastole
5: Diameter of LV in diastole
6: Diameter of LV in systole

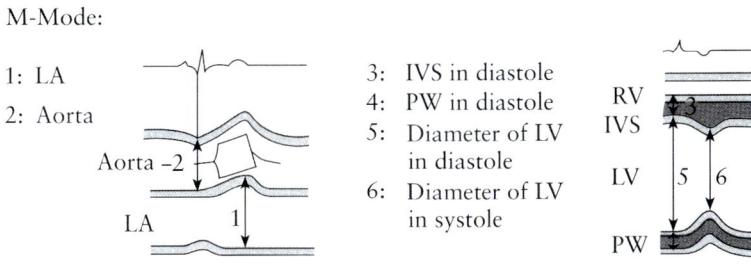

Figure A1.1 Sites for making 2D or M-mode measurements. Published normal ranges are calculated using measurements made from leading edge to leading edge. Recent guidelines suggest measuring from inner to inner. Diastolic measurements are timed with the onset of the QRS complex of the electrocardiogram and left ventricular (LV) systolic measurements at peak septal deflection when septal motion is normal or at peak posterior wall (PW) deflection when septal motion is abnormal. Left atrial (LA) diameter is taken as the maximum possible at the end of ventricular systole. IVS, interventricular septum; RV, right ventricle

Table A1.1 Normal intracardiac dimensions (cm) in men and women aged 18–72 years, 150–203 cm (59–80 in) in height[1,2]

	Men	**Women**
LA	3.0–4.5 ($n = 288$)	2.7–4.0 ($n = 524$)
LVDD	4.3–5.9 ($n = 394$)	4.0–5.2 ($n = 643$)
LVSD	2.6–4.0 ($n = 288$)	2.3–3.5 ($n = 524$)
IVS (diastole)	0.6–1.3 ($n = 106$)	0.5–1.2 ($n = 109$)
PW (diastole)	0.6–1.2 ($n = 106$)	0.5–1.1 ($n = 119$)

LLA, left atrium; LVDD, left ventricular diastolic dimension; LVSD, left ventricular systolic dimension; IVS, interventricular septum; PW, posterior wall

Table A1.2 Upper limit of intracardiac dimensions (cm) by height (m)[1,3]

	Height									
	1.41–1.45	1.46–1.50	1.51–1.55	1.56–1.60	1.61–1.65	1.66–1.70	1.71–1.75	1.76–1.80	1.81–1.85	1.86–1.90
M-mode										
Male										
LVDD			5.3	5.4	5.5	5.5	5.6	5.7	5.8	5.9
LVSD			3.6	3.7	3.7	3.8	3.8	3.9	3.9	4.0
Female										
LVDD	4.9	4.9	5.0	5.1	5.1	5.2	5.3	5.3		
LVSD	3.1	3.2	3.3	3.3	3.4	3.4	3.5	3.5		
2D										
Ann	2.0	2.0	2.1	2.1	2.2	2.2	2.3	2.3	2.4	2.4
LA	3.2	3.3	3.4	3.4	3.5	3.6	3.6	3.7	3.8	3.9

LVDD, left ventricular diastolic dimension; LVSD, left ventricular systolic dimension; Ann, aortic annulus; LA, left atrium

Appendices

Table A1.3 Intracardiac dimensions (cm) on 2D echocardiography by body surface area (BSA)[a,4]

		BSA (m^2)		
		1.4–1.6	1.6–1.8	1.8–2.0
1. Parasternal long-axis	Diastole	3.4–4.9	3.6–5.1	3.9–5.3
	Systole	2.3–3.9	2.4–4.1	2.5–4.4
2. Parasternal short-axis, mitral level	Diastole	3.7–5.4	3.9–5.7	4.1–6.0
	Systole	2.6–4.0	2.8–4.3	2.9–4.4
3. Parasternal short-axis, papillary	Diastole	3.5–5.5	3.8–5.8	4.1–6.1
	Systole	2.3–3.9	2.4–4.0	2.6–4.1
4. 4-chamber mediolateral	Diastole	3.9–5.4	4.0–5.6	4.1–5.9
	Systole	2.7–4.5	2.9–4.7	3.1–4.9
5. 4-chamber long-axis	Diastole	5.9–8.3	6.3–8.7	6.6–9.0
	Systole	4.5–6.9	4.6–7.4	4.6–7.9

[a]See Figure A1.2 for measurement sites

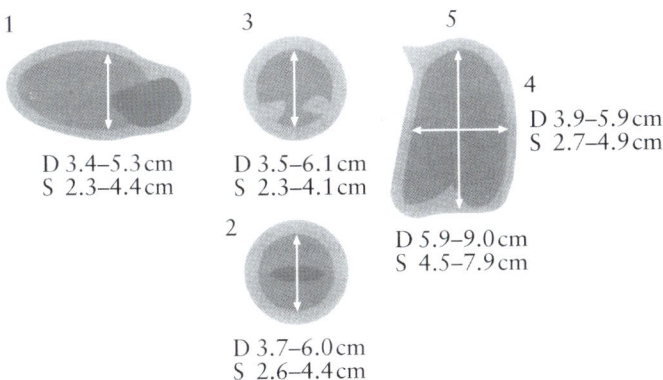

Figure A1.2 Sites for making 2D measurements. D, diastole; S, systole

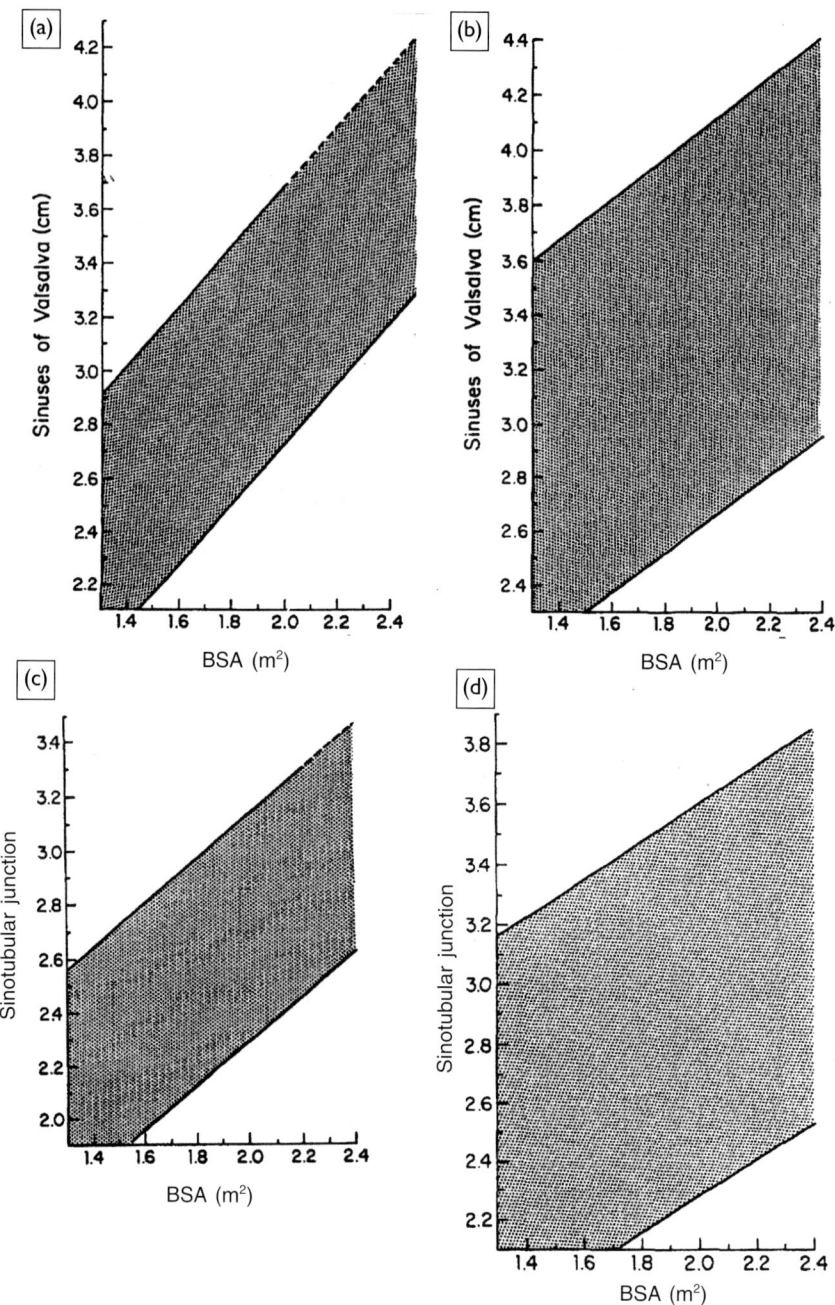

Figure A1.3 Aortic dimensions by body surface area (BSA). (a,b) 95% range at the sinus of valsalva for adults aged under 40 (a), and adults aged 40 years and over (b). (c,d) 95% range at the sinotubular junction for adults aged under 40 (c) and adults aged 40 years and over (d). (Reproduced from Roman MJ et al. Am J Cardiol 1989; 64:507–12[18] with permission from Elsevier)

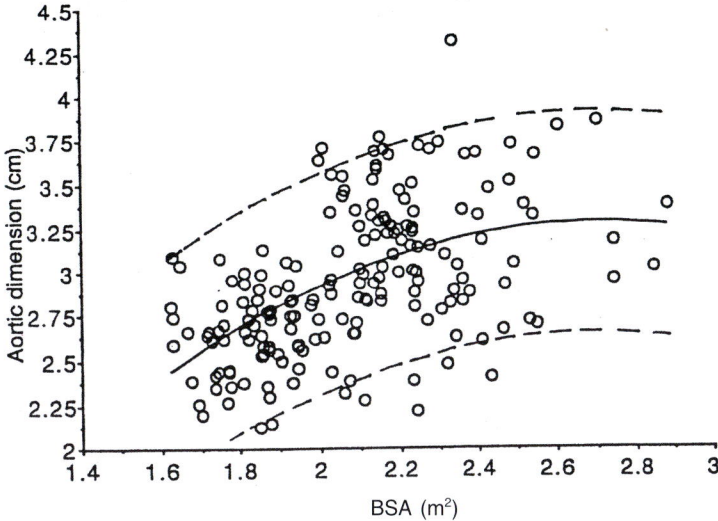

Figure A1.4 Aortic dimension at the sinotubular junction in tall subjects. The measurements displayed here were made using M-mode, which is no longer recommended, but may give a guide to the significance of 2D measurements (Reproduced from Reed et al. Am J Cardiol 1993; 71:608–10[19] with permission from Elsevier)

Table A1.4 Right-sided dimensions[5,6]

	Systole	Diastole
Maximal width in 4-chamber (cm)	3.6	4.3
Length in 4-chamber (cm)	8.1	9.1
Width in parasternal short-axis (cm)	3.4	3.8
Width in parasternal long-axis (cm)		3.0
Width in parasternal modified long-axis (cm)		5.4
Right ventricular outflow parasternal short-axis (cm)		3.2

Table A1.5 Normal ranges for measures of diastolic function[7–9]

Mitral valve E (m/s)	0.4–1.0	0.3–0.9 (elderly)
Mitral valve A (m/s)	0.2–0.6	0.3–0.9 (elderly)
E/A ratio	0.7–3.1	0.5–1.7 (elderly)
Mitral E deceleration time (ms)	139–219	138–282 (elderly)
Isovolumic relaxation time (IVRT) (ms)	54–98	56–124 (elderly)

2. NORMAL VALUES FOR REPLACEMENT HEART VALVES[10,12]

- Surprisingly few published data exist for normally functioning valves. These tables draw on all the literature to the end of 2005.
- The short and long forms of the modified Bernoulli equation and the classical and modified versions of the continuity equation are used variously, and this accounts for some variation in results.
- Pressure half-time and the Hatle formula are not valid in normally functioning mitral prostheses, and are omitted.
- Doppler results are broadly similar for valves sharing a similar design. For simplicity, results for one design in each category are given, with a list of other valve designs for which data exist.
- Sizing conventions vary, so it is possible that a given label size for a valve not on the list may not be equivalent to those that are. A change on serial studies is more revealing than a single measurement, and the echocardiogram must be interpreted in the clinical context.
- The values (Tables A2.1–A2.3) shown are means, with standard deviation in parentheses.

3. SUMMARY OF FORMULAE

3.1 Bernoulli equation

This equates potential and kinetic energy up- and downstream from a stenosis. The modified formula is used in two forms:

short modified Bernoulli equation

$$\Delta P = 4v_2^2$$

long modified Bernoulli equation

$$\Delta P = 4(v_2^2 - v_1^2)$$

where ΔP is the transvalvar pressure difference, v_1 is the subvalvar velocity, and v_2 is the transvalvar velocity. The short form can be used when the subvalvar velocity is much less than the transvalvar velocity, e.g., in mitral stenosis or moderate or severe aortic stenosis (v_2 >3 m/s), but *not* in mild aortic stenosis or for normally functioning replacement valves.

3.2 Continuity equation

This is used in two forms:

classical continuity equation

$$EOA = CSA \times \frac{VTI_1}{VTI_2}$$

Table A2.1 Aortic position: biological

	V_{max} (m/s)	Peak ΔP (mmHg)	Mean ΔP (mmHg)	EOA (cm^2)
Stented porcine: *Carpentier–Edwards standard as example (values similar for Carpentier–Edwards Supra-Annular, Intact, Hancock I and II, Mosaic, Biocor, Epic)*				
19 mm		43.5 (12.7)	25.6 (8.0)	0.9 (0.2)
21 mm	2.8 (0.5)	27.2 (7.6)	17.3 (6.2)	1.5 (0.3)
23 mm	2.8 (0.7)	28.9 (7.5)	16.1 (6.2)	1.7 (0.5)
25 mm	2.6 (0.6)	24.0 (7.1)	12.9 (4.6)	1.9 (0.5)
27 mm	2.5 (0.5)	22.1 (8.2)	12.1 (5.5)	2.3 (0.6)
29 mm	2.4 (0.4)		9.9 (2.9)	2.8 (0.5)
Stented bovine pericardial: *Baxter Perimount as example (similar for Mitroflow, Edwards Pericardial, Labcor-Santiago, Mitroflow)*				
19 mm	2.8 (0.1)	32.5 (8.5)	19.5 (5.5)	1.3 (0.2)
21 mm	2.6 (0.4)	24.9 (7.7)	13.8 (4.0)	1.3 (0.3)
23 mm	2.3 (0.5)	19.9 (7.4)	11.5 (3.9)	1.6 (0.3)
25 mm	2.0 (0.3)	16.5 (7.8)	10.7 (3.8)	1.6 (0.4)
27 mm		12.8 (5.4)	4.8 (2.2)	2.0 (0.4)
Homograft				
22 mm	1.7 (0.3)		5.8 (3.2)	2.0 (0.6)
26 mm	1.4 (0.6)		6.8 (2.9)	2.4 (0.7)
Stentless				
Whole root as inclusion: St Jude Toronto (similar for Prima)				
21 mm		22.6 (14.5)	10.7 (7.2)	1.3 (0.6)
23 mm		16.2 (9.0)	8.2 (4.7)	1.6 (0.6)
25 mm		12.7 (8.2)	6.3 (4.1)	1.8 (0.5)
27 mm		10.1 (5.8)	5.0 (2.9)	2.0 (0.3)
29 mm		7.7 (4.4)	4.1 (2.4)	2.4 (0.6)
Cryolife–O'Brien (similar for Freestyle)				
19 mm			9.0 (2.0)	1.5 (0.3)
21 mm			6.6 (2.9)	1.7 (0.4)
23 mm			6.0 (2.3)	2.3 (0.2)
25 mm			6.1 (2.6)	2.6 (0.2)
27 mm			4.0 (2.4)	2.8 (0.3)

V_{max}, peak velocity; ΔP, pressure difference; EOA, effective orifice area

Table A2.2 Aortic position: Mechanical

	V_{max} (m/s)	Peak ΔP (mmHg)	Mean ΔP (mmHg)	EOA (cm^2)
Single tilting disk				
Medtronic-Hall (values similar for Bjork–Shiley Monostrut and CC, Omnicarbon, Omniscience)				
20 mm	2.9 (0.4)	34.4 (13.1)	17.1 (5.3)	1.2 (0.5)
21 mm	2.4 (0.4)	26.9 (10.5)	14.1 (5.9)	1.1 (0.2)
23 mm	2.4 (0.6)	26.9 (8.9)	13.5 (4.8)	1.4 (0.4)
25 mm	2.3 (0.5)	17.1 (7.0)	9.5 (4.3)	1.5 (0.5)
27 mm	2.1 (0.5)	18.9 (9.7)	8.7 (5.6)	1.9 (0.2)
Bileaflet mechanical				
Intrannular: St Jude Standard (similar for Carbomedics Standard, Edwards Mira, ATS, Sorin Bicarbon)				
19 mm	2.9 (0.5)	35.2 (11.2)	19.0 (6.3)	1.0 (0.2)
21 mm	2.6 (0.5)	28.3 (10.0)	15.8 (5.7)	1.3 (0.3)
23 mm	2.6 (0.4)	25.3 (7.9)	13.8 (5.3)	1.6 (0.4)
25 mm	2.4 (0.5)	22.6 (7.7)	12.7 (5.1)	1.9 (0.5)
27 mm	2.2 (0.4)	19.9 (7.6)	11.2 (4.8)	2.4 (0.6)
29 mm	2.0 (0.1)	17.7 (6.4)	9.9 (2.9)	2.8 (0.6)
Intra-annular modified cuff or partially supra-annular: MCRI On-X (similar for St Jude Regent, St Jude HP, Carbmedics Reduced Cuff, Medtronic Advantage)				
19 mm		21.3 (10.8)	11.8 (3.4)	1.5 (0.2)
21 mm		16.4 (5.9)	9.9 (3.6)	1.7 (0.4)
23 mm		15.9 (6.4)	8.6 (3.4)	1.9 (0.6)
25 mm		16.5 (10.2)	6.9 (4.3)	2.4 (0.6)
Supra-annular: *Carbomedics TopHat*				
21 mm	2.6 (0.4)	30.2 (10.9)	14.9 (5.4)	1.2 (0.3)
23 mm	2.4 (0.6)	24.2 (7.6)	12.5 (4.4)	1.4 (0.4)
25 mm			9.5 (2.9)	1.6 (0.3)
Ball and cage: *Starr–Edwards*				
23 mm	3.4 (0.6)	32.6 (12.8)	22.0 (9.0)	1.1 (0.2)
24 mm	3.6 (0.5)	34.1 (10.3)	22.1 (7.5)	1.1 (0.3)
26 mm	3.0 (0.2)	31.8 (9.0)	19.7 (6.1)	
27 mm		30.8 (6.3)	18.5 (3.7)	
29 mm		29.3 (9.3)	16.3 (5.5)	

V_{max}, peak velocity; ΔP, pressure difference; EOA, effective orifice area

Table A2.3 Mitral position

	V_{max} (m/s)	Mean ΔP (mmHg)
Stented Porcine: *Carpentier–Edwards (values similar for Intact, Hancock)*		
27 mm		6.0 (2.0)
29 mm	1.5 (0.3)	4.7 (2.0)
31 mm	1.5 (0.3)	4.5 (2.0)
33 mm	1.4 (0.2)	5.4 (4.0)
Pericardial: *Ionescu–Shiley (similar for Labcor–Santiago, Hancock Pericardial, Carpentier–Edwards Pericardial)*		
25 mm	1.4 (0.2)	4.9 (1.1)
27 mm	1.3 (0.2)	3.2 (0.8)
29 mm	1.4 (0.2)	3.2 (0.6)
31 mm	1.3 (0.1)	2.7 (0.4)
Single tilting disc: *Bjork–Shiley Monostrut (similar for Omnicarbon)*		
25 mm	1.8 (0.3)	5.6 (2.3)
27 mm	1.7 (0.4)	4.5 (2.2)
29 mm	1.6 (0.3)	4.3 (1.6)
31 mm	1.7 (0.3)	4.9 (1.6)
33 mm	1.3 (0.3)	
Bileaflet: *Carbomedics (similar for St Jude)*		
25 mm	1.6 (0.2)	4.3 (0.7)
27 mm	1.6 (0.3)	3.7 (1.5)
29 mm	1.8 (0.3)	3.7 (1.3)
31 mm	1.6 (0.4)	3.3 (1.1)
33 mm	1.4 (0.3)	3.4 (1.5)
Caged ball: *Starr–Edwards*		
28 mm	1.8 (0.2)	7.0 (2.8)
30 mm	1.8 (0.2)	7.0 (2.5)
32 mm	1.9 (0.4)	5.1 (2.5)

V_{max}, peak velocity; ΔP, pressure difference

modified continuity equation

$$EOA = CSA \times \frac{v_1}{v_2}$$

where EOA is the effective orifice area, CSA is the cross-sectional area of the left ventricular outflow tract, and VTI_1 and VTI_2 are the subaortic and transaortic systolic velocity time integrals. The modified form is only a reasonable approximation in significant aortic stenosis.

3.3 Pressure half-time

The pressure half-time orifice area formula gives the effective mitral orifice area MOA (in cm²)

$$MOA = \frac{220}{T_{1/2}}$$

where $T_{1/2}$ is the pressure half-time (in ms). This formula should only be used in moderate or severe stenosis. It is not valid for normally functioning replacement valves.

3.4 Stroke volume

The stroke volume SV is given by

$$SV = CSA \times VTI_1$$

where CSA is the cross-sectional area of the left ventricular outflow tract (in cm²), and VTI_1 is the subaortic velocity time integral (in cm).

3.5 Shunt calculation

The stroke volume is calculated for the aortic valve as above and then for the pulmonary valve using the diameter at the pulmonary annulus and the velocity time integral calculated with the pulsed sample at the level of the annulus. If the annulus cannot be imaged reliably, the diameter of the pulmonary artery and the level for velocity recording should be taken downstream. The shunt is then the ratio of pulmonary stroke volume to aortic stroke volume (see also Table 11.2)

3.6 Flow

The flow is given by

$$Flow = CSA \times VTI_1 \times \frac{1000}{SET}$$

where CSA is the cross-sectional area of the left ventricular outflow tract (in cm^2), VTI$_1$ is the subaortic velocity time integral (in cm), and SET is the systolic ejection time (from opening to closing artefact of the aortic signal) (in ms).

3.7 LV mass

The left ventricular mass is given by

$$\text{LV mass} = 1.04 \times [(\text{LVDD} + \text{IVS} + \text{PW})^3 - \text{LVDD}^3] - 13.6$$

where LVD is the LV internal diameter, IVS is the thickness of the interventricular septum, and LPW is the thickness of the LV posterior wall. This is the Devereux formula, which is widely applied although it is not as accurate as two-dimensional methods. It also uses the Penn convention of measurement, taking the septal and posterior wall thicknesses from inner to inner. Using the ASE convention (i.e. leading edge to leading edge), the simplified and modified formula is

$$\text{LV mass} = 0.83 \times [(\text{LVDD} + \text{IVS} + \text{PW})^3 - \text{LVDD}^3]$$

3.8 Other formulae

These are either not in universal use or lack adequate validation data

3.9 Systemic vascular resistance from mitral regurgitation and stroke distance

- Measure the peak velocity of the mitral regurgitant signal on continuous wave: MR V_{max}.
- Measure the stroke distance in the apical 5-chamber view: VTI$_1$.
- The systemic vascular resistance is then[13]

$$\frac{\text{MR } V_{max}}{\text{VTI}_1}$$

- A ratio >0.27 suggests high resistance and <0.2 suggests normal resistance.

3.10 Mean pulmonary artery pressure from pulmonary regurgitant signal

This could be useful if an estimate of pulmonary pressure is needed and there is no measurable tricuspid regurgitant jet.

- Measure the peak pulmonary regurgitant velocity: PR V_{max}.

- The mean pulmonary artery pressure is $4 \times PR\ V_{max}^2$, with no need to add an estimate of right atrial pressure.[14]

3.11 RV systolic function using the Tei index[15]

- Record the transtricuspid flow using pulsed Doppler. Measure the time a from the end of one signal to the start of the next.
- Record the transpulmonary flow using pulsed Doppler. Measure the ejection time b, which is the time from the start to the end of flow.
- The Tei index is then $(a - b)/b$.
- The normal range for the right ventricle is 0.2–0.32.

3.12 Grading aortic stenosis from the continuous-wave signal

The ratio of peak to mean gradient has been shown to correlate well with effective orifice area by the continuity equation in patients with both normal and reduced LV ejection fraction[16] and could be a guide to the need for dobutamine stress in patients with a low LV ejection fraction and aortic stenosis of uncertain grade.

- Trace the optimum continuous wave signal to derive peak and mean gradient.
- The ratio of the peak to mean gradient is then interpreted as shown in Table A3.1.

Table A3.1 Interpretation of peak to mean gradient ratio

Ratio	Grade of aortic stenosis
<1.5	Always severe
1.5–1.7	Severe stenosis possible; consider dobutamine stress
>1.7	Mild or moderate

3.13 LV diastolic function using flow propagation[17]

- From a 4-chamber view, place the colour box over the mitral valve and the base of the LV. Place the cursor over the inflow signal. Reduce the velocity on the colour scale if necessary to ensure a clear aliasing signal in the red forward flow on colour M-mode.
- Use the calliper to draw a line about 4–5 cm long along the edge of the colour change on the early diastolic signal and calculate the slope (V_p).
- Divide this into the peak transmitral E-wave velocity.
- High filling pressures are suggested by a V_p/E ratio >1.8.

4. BODY SURFACE NOMOGRAM

See Figure A4.1.

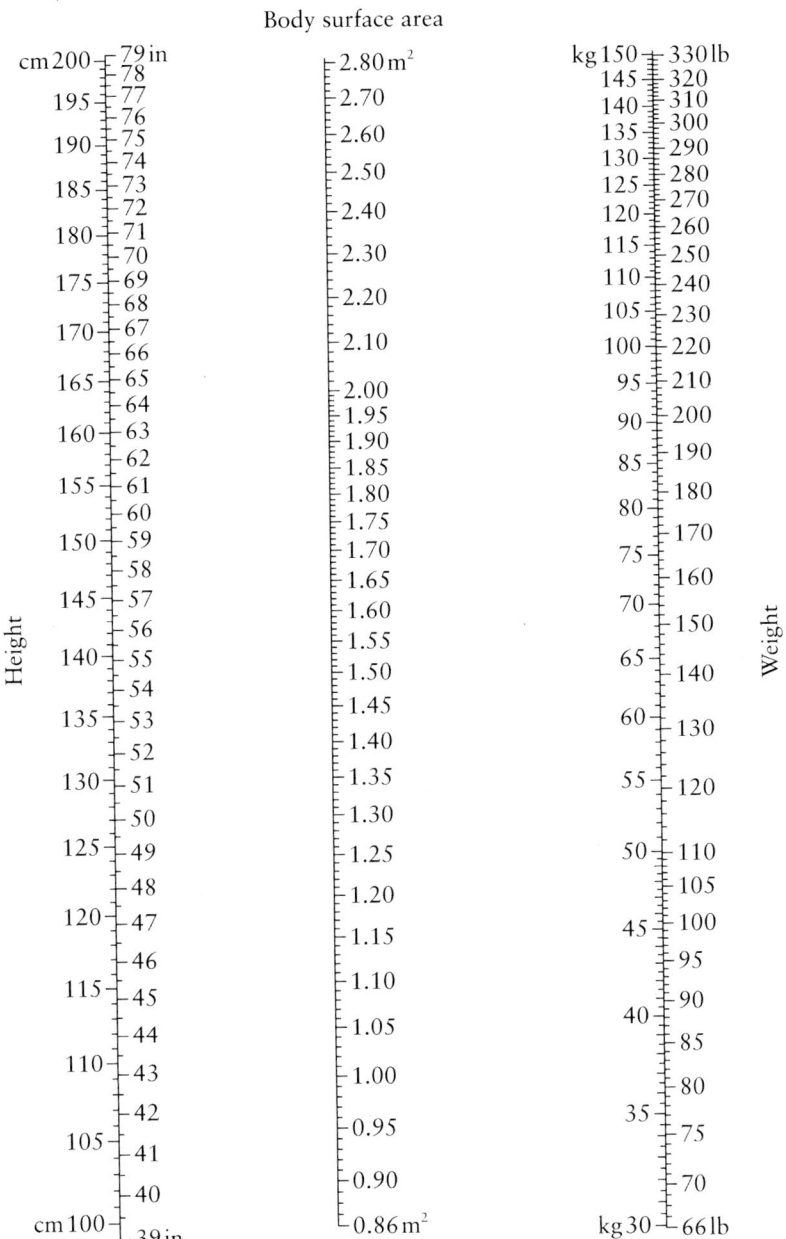

Figure A4.1 Body surface nomogram. Put a straight edge against the patient's height and weight, and read off the body surface area on the middle column

REFERENCES

1. Lauer MS, Larson MG, Levy D. Gender-specific reference M-mode values in adults: population-derived values with consideration of the impact of height. J Am Coll Cardiol 1995; 26:1039–46.
2. Devereux RB, Lutas EM, Casale PN, et al. Standardization of M-mode echocardiographic left ventricular anatomic measurements. J Am Coll Cardiol 1984; 4:1222–30.
3. Nidorf SM, Picard MH, Triulzi MO, et al. New perspectives in the assessment of cardiac chamber dimensions during development and adulthood. J Am Coll Cardiol 1992; 19:983–988.
4. Pearlman JD, Triulzi MO, King ME, Newell J, Weyman AE. Limits of normal left ventricular dimensions in growth and development: analysis of dimensions and variance in the two-dimensional echocardiograms of 268 normal healthy subjects. J Am Coll Cardiol 1988; 12:1432–41.
5. Triulzi MO, Gillam LD, Gentile F. Normal adult cross-sectional echocardiographic values: linear dimensions and chamber areas. Echocardiography 1984; 1:403–26.
6. Foale R, Nihoyannopoulos P, McKenna W, et al. Echocardiographic measurement of the normal adult right ventricle. Br Heart J 1986; 56:33–44.
7. Zarich SW, Arbuckle BE, Cohen LR, Roberts M, Nesto RW. Diastolic abnormalities in young asymptomatic diabetic patients assessed by pulsed Doppler echocardiography. J Am Coll Cardiol 1988; 12:114–20.
8. Van Dam I, Fast J, de Boo T, et al. Normal diastolic filling patterns of the left ventricle. Eur Heart J 1988; 9:165–71.
9. Sagie A, Benjamin EJ, Galderisi M, et al. Reference values for Doppler indexes of left ventricular diastolic filling in the elderly. J Am Soc Echocardiogr 1993; 6:570–6.
10. Wang Z, Grainger N, Chambers J. Doppler echocardiography in normally functioning replacement heart valves: a literature review. J Heart Valve Dis 1995; 4:591–614.
11. Rajani R, Mukherjee D, Chambers J. Doppler echocardiography in normally functioning replacement aortic valves: a literature review. In preparation 2006.
12. Rosenhek R, Binder T, Maurer G, Baumgartner H. Normal values for Doppler echocardiographic assessment of heart valve prostheses. J Am Soc Echocardiogr 2003 16:1116–27.
13. Abbas AE, Fortuin FD, Patel B, et al. Noninvasive measurement of systemic vascular resistance using Doppler echocardiography. J Am Soc Echocardiogr 2004; 17:834–8.
14. Masuyama T, Kodama K, Kitabatake A, et al. Continuous-wave Doppler echocardiographic detection of pulmonary regurgitation and its application to noninvasive estimation of pulmonary artery pressure. Circulation 1986; 74:484–92.
15. Tei C, Dujardin KS, Hodge DO, et al. Doppler echocardiographic index for assessment of global right ventricular function. J Am Soc Echocardiogr 1996; 9:838–47.
16. Chambers J, Rajani R, Hankins M, Cook R. The peak to mean pressure decrease ratio: a new method of assessing aortic stenosis. J Am Soc Echocardiogr 2005; 18:674–8.
17. Takatsuji H, Mikami T, Urasawa K, et al. A new approach for evaluation of left ventricular diastolic function: spatial and temporal analysis of left ventricular filling flow propagation by color M-mode Doppler echocardiography. J Am Coll Cardiol 1996; 27:365–71.
18. Roman MJ, Devereux RB, Kramer-Fox R, O'Loughlin J. Two-dimensional echocardiographic aortic root dimensions in normal children and adults. Am J Cardiol 1989; 64:507–12.
19. Reed CM, Rickey PA, Pullian DA, Somes GW. Aortic dimensions in tall men and women. Am J Cardiol 1993; 71:608–10.

INDEX

Page numbers in *italics* indicate figures or tables.

amyloid 29, *34*
  vs hypertrophic cardiomyopathy 33
aneurysms, true *vs* false 24, *25*, *26*
angiosarcoma 116
aorta 79–85
  aortic valve disease 41, 42
  calcification 82
  checklist for reporting 84
  coarctation *see* coarctation of aorta
  diameters 79, *80*, *81*, *132*, *133*
  flow reversal at arch 42, *44*, *45*, *46*
  relations, congenital disease 102
aortic annulus *130*
aortic dilatation 79–80, *80*
aortic dissection 82, *82*–3, *84*
aortic prosthetic valves 67–70
  normal values 134, *135–6*
  obstruction 70, *70*
  regurgitation 67–8, *69*, *71*
aortic regurgitation 42–6
  acute 42, 77
  aetiology *43*
  colour flow mapping 42, *43*, *44*
  endocarditis 77
  flow reversal at arch 42, *44*, *45*, *46*
  severity grading 46, *46*
  vena contracta width 42, *46*
aortic stenosis 39–41
  clues to aetiology *39*
  Doppler measurements 39–40
  grading from continuous-wave signal 40, 140, *140*
  low flow 41, *41*
  RV dilatation and 91
  severity assessment 40, *40*
aortic valve
  appearance 39, *39*, 42
  bicuspid 79, 80, *80*
  effective orifice area (EOA) 40, *40*
  surgery, aortic examination before 80–2
  thickening with no stenosis 40
arrhythmogenic right ventricular dysplasia (ARVD) 35–6, *36*, 90
arterial paradox *16*, 112
arterial territories, heart *6*
arteriosclerotic dilatation of aorta 79, *80*
ASD *see* atrial septal defect
athletic heart 28, *28*
  vs hypertrophic cardiomyopathy 32, 33
atria 87–8
  assessment in congenital disease 102
  bilateral enlargement 88
  thrombus 49, 116
atrial fibrillation *122*
atrial septal defect (ASD) 99, *100*, 104
  post-procedure studies *106*, 107
  primum 99, *99*
  RV dilatation 90, 93
  secundum 99
  TOE before device closure 99, *101*
atrioventricular septal defect (AVSD) *104*, 106
atrioventricular (AV) valves 102
  common *104*
A wave
  pulmonary vein (PV) *14*
  transmitral 11, *11*, 13, *133*

Bernoulli equation 134
biatrial enlargement 88
body surface area (BSA)
    aortic dimensions by 132
    intracardiac dimensions by 131
    nomogram 141

cardiac arrest 119
cardiac output 8
cardiac resynchronisation therapy 17–19
cardiac surgery, hypotension after 113, 121
cardiomyopathies 27–37
clinical advice, indications for urgent 125
clinical requests, specific 119–24
coarctation of aorta 80, 83–5, 84
    post-repair/stenting study 106, 107
cocaine 123
congenital disease, adult 99–108
    post-procedure studies 106, 107, 107, 108
    simple defects 99–100
    suspicious findings 102
    systematic study 100–7
continuity equation 134–8
contrast echocardiography, indications 125
coronary sinus, dilated 105, 107

dilated cardiomyopathy 27–9
dimensions, normal intracardiac 129–33
discordant connections 102
dobutamine stress echocardiography 41

E/A ratio, transmitral 13, 15, 133
E deceleration time, transmitral 11, 11, 13, 15, 133
E/E' ratio, transmitral 12, 13
Ehlers–Danlos syndrome 79, 80, 83, 84
ejection fraction (EF)
    left ventricle 7, 7, 23
    right ventricle 91

embolism, peripheral 122
emergency echocardiography 119–20
endocarditis 75–8
    indications for TOE 77, 77
    local complications 75, 75–6, 76
    Loeffler's 35
    LV assessment 77
    predisposing abnormalities 77, 77
    valve destruction 76
    vegetations 75, 76
endomyocardial fibrosis 35
E' velocity 12, 13
E wave, transmitral 11, 11, 12, 13, 133

Fabry's disease 34
Fallot's tetralogy, post-repair study 107, 107
flow 138–9
formulae 134–40
fractional shortening (FS) 5
    aortic regurgitation 42
    mitral regurgitation 57–8

glycogen storage disease 34

haemochromatosis 29, 34
Hatle formula 47
heart failure 122
    with apparently normal LV 33, 33
HIV infection 123
hypertension 124
    vs hypertrophic cardiomyopathy 32, 32
hypertrophic cardiomyopathy 29–33
    apical 30
    obstructive 31
    vs amyloid 33
    vs athletic heart 32, 33
    vs hypertension 32, 32
hypotension
    after cardiac surgery 113, 121
    after invasive procedures 119, 120

inferior vena cava (IVC)
    engorged 111
    estimation of RA pressure from 94, 94

masses 116
relations, congenital disease 102
interventricular delay, cardiac resynchronisation 18
interventricular septum (IVS) 31, *129*
intra-left ventricular (LV) delay, cardiac resynchronisation 18–19
isovolumic relaxation time (IVRT) *133*

left atrial (LA) dilatation 87, *87*
  LV diastolic function and 11
  mitral regurgitation 57
  mitral stenosis 49
left atrium (LA)
  assessment of size 87, *87*
  dimensions *129, 130*
  masses 116
  relations, congenital disease 102
left ventricle (LV) 5–21
  anatomic/morphologic 102
  apex, abnormal thickening 35
  ejection fraction (EF) 7, *7*, 23
  fractional shortening *see* fractional shortening
  hyperkinetic/hyperdynamic *28*, 42, 57
  hypokinetic *27, 28*, 39
  masses 116, *116, 117*
  regional wall thickness (RWT) 30
  volume load 100
left ventricular (LV) cavity dimensions 5
  aortic regurgitation 42
  cardiomyopathies 27–8, 30
  endocarditis 77
  mitral regurgitation 57–8
  normal ranges *129, 130*
left ventricular (LV) cavity volumes 7
left ventricular (LV) diastolic function 10, 11–13, *14*
  diagnosis of dysfunction 13, *13*
  flow propagation method 140
  hypertrophic cardiomyopathy 31
  mitral filling pattern 11, *11*, 14
  normal ranges *133*
  PV flow 13, *14*

restrictive filling 13, *13*
tissue Doppler *12*, 13
left ventricular (LV) dilatation 27, 27–9, *28*
left ventricular (LV) function
  aortic dissection 83
  aortic regurgitation 42
  aortic stenosis 39
  cardiac resynchronisation therapy 17–18
  endocarditis 77
  mitral regurgitation 8, *9*, 57–8
  see also left ventricular (LV) diastolic function; left ventricular (LV) systolic function
left ventricular (LV) hypertrophy 29–33, *30*
  concentric 30, *31*
  diastolic function and 11
  grading *31*
  see also hypertrophic cardiomyopathy
left ventricular (LV) mass 30, *31*, 139
left ventricular (LV) non-compaction *35*, 35–6, *36*
left ventricular (LV) outflow tract
  acceleration 31
  radius 8
left ventricular (LV) systolic diameter 42, 57–8
left ventricular (LV) systolic function 5–11
  cardiomyopathies 27–8, 31
  dP/dt 8, *8, 9*
  global 7–8, 23
  long-axis 9, *9, 10*
  mitral regurgitation 57–8
  regional wall motion 5, *5, 6*, 23
  wall motion index 5
left ventricular (LV) systolic volume 58
Loeffler's endocarditis 35
lupus erythematosus, systemic *124*

Marfan syndrome 79, *80*, 83, 84

masses 115–17
  attached to valves 115, *115*
  description *76*, 115
  extrinsic *117*
  haemodynamic effect 117
  LA or RA 116, *116*
  LV or RV 116, *116, 117*
measurements
  minimum set 2
  normal ranges 129–33
  reporting 2–3
minimum standard echocardiogram 1–2
mitral orifice area (MOA) 138
  by planimetry 47, *47, 48*
mitral prosthetic valves 70–2
  normal values 134, *137*
  obstruction 72, *72*
  regurgitation 70
mitral regurgitation 49–58
  aetiology *51*
  after myocardial infarction 23, 24, *24*
  colour flow mapping 53–5, *54, 56*
  continuous wave signal 55
  functional 55
  grading *52, 57*
  LV function 8, *9, 57–8*
  pulsed Doppler 55–7
  systemic vascular resistance from 139
mitral stenosis 46–9, *50*
  markers of successful balloon valvotomy 49, *49, 50, 51*
  RV dilatation 48, *91*
  severity assessment 48, *48*
mitral valve
  appearance and movement 46–7, *49, 52*
  filling patterns 11, *11, 14*
  myocardial infarction 23
  prolapse 49, *52, 54*
  repair 57, 58, *58*
  restricted leaflet motion 49, *52, 55, 56*
  segments *53*
M-mode measurements 2, *129, 130*
murmurs, unknown cause *123*

Mustard–Senning procedures 107, *107, 108*
myocardial infarction 23–6
  complications 24, *24, 25, 26*
  right ventricle 23, 90

nomogram, body surface *141*
normal values
  cardiac dimensions 129–33
  replacement heart valves 134, *135–7*

paradox, arterial *16*, 112
patent ductus arteriosus (PDA) 100, *100, 103*
  post-closure studies *106*, 107
patent foramen ovale (PFO), post-closure studies *106*, 107
pericardial constriction
  arterial paradox *16*
  vs restrictive cardiomyopathy *15*, 15–17
pericardial effusion 109–13
  size and distribution *109*, 109–11
  vs pleural effusion *109, 110*
pericardial region, causes of abnormal *112*
pericardiocentesis 111, *113*
pericarditis, effusive–constrictive 113
pleural effusion *109, 110*
posterior wall (PW) *129*
pressure half-time 138
prosthetic valves 65–73
  aortic position 67–70, *135–6*
  appearance 65, *65–7, 66*
  biological 65, *66*, 66–7
  checklist for reporting *69*
  endocarditis 75
  indications for TOE 67, *68*, 70
  LV and RV function and PA pressure 67
  mechanical 65, *66, 67*
  mitral position 70–2, *137*
  normal values 134, *135–7*
  regurgitation or obstruction 67, *69*
  right-sided 72
pseudoaneurysms, *vs* true aneurysms 24, *25, 26*

pulmonary and aortic flow, delay between 18
pulmonary artery (PA)
  assessment, congenital disease 102–5
  dimensions 83
  velocity 96, 97
pulmonary artery (PA) pressure
  adult congenital disease 105
  aortic stenosis 41
  diastolic, estimating 94, 95
  mean, from pulmonary regurgitant signal 139–40
  mitral stenosis 48, 48
  patent ductus arteriosus 100
  pulmonary valve disease 63
  systolic, estimating 94, 94
pulmonary embolism, massive 120
pulmonary hypertension 94–8
  causes 96, 96
  detection in absence of tricuspid regurgitation 94–6, 97
  mitral regurgitation 57
  RV dilatation 90, 91
pulmonary regurgitation 61–3, 62
  mean PA pressure from 139–40
  PA diastolic pressure estimation 94, 95
  RV dilatation 90
pulmonary stenosis 61–3
pulmonary valve 61–3
  appearance 61
  pressure difference across 63
  prostheses 72, 73

radiation injury 34
regional wall thickness (RWT) 30
renal failure, chronic 124
replacement heart valves *see* prosthetic valves
reports, echocardiography 2–4
requests, specific clinical 119–24
restrictive cardiomyopathy 33–4, 34
  vs pericardial constriction 15, 15–17
right atrium (RA)
  dilatation 87, 87, 88
  masses 116, 116

pressure estimation 94, 94
relations, congenital disease 102
right heart 89–98
  dimensions 133
right ventricle (RV) 89–94
  diastolic collapse 111
  ejection fraction 91
  hypertrophy 91
  infarction 23, 90
  masses 116, 116, 117
  relations, congenital disease 102
  size estimation 89, 90
  systolic function 91, 91, 92, 140
  systolic pressure 94
right ventricular (RV) dilatation 89, 89–93
  active 90, 90
  adult congenital disease 105
  causes 90, 90
  hypokinetic 90, 90
  isolated 35
  left-sided disease 48, 91

sarcoid 28, 29, 34
semilunar valves 102
septal to posterior wall delay on M-mode 18
shunt calculation 99, 100, 100, 138
shunts, intracardiac 105
Simpson's rule 7
spectral Doppler, minimum standard 2
standard echocardiogram, minimum 1–2
stress echocardiography 41, 127
stroke 122
stroke distance 7–8, 139
stroke volume (SV) 8, 138
subaortic velocity time integral (VTI1) 7, 7–8
sum asynchrony time 18
superior vena cava (SVC), left-sided 105, 107
systemic lupus erythematosus 124
systemic vascular resistance 139

tamponade, signs 111, 112
Tei index 140

tetralogy of Fallot, post-repair study 107, *107*
thrombus *24*, 29
  intra-atrial 49, 116
  intraventricular 116
  IVC 116
tissue Doppler
  interventricular delay 18
  left ventricle *12*, 13, 17
  right ventricle 91, *91*, *93*
TOE *see* transoesophageal echocardiography
transient ischaemic attack (TIA) 122
transmitral duration 13
transoesophageal echocardiography (TOE)
  adult congenital disease 99, *101*
  aortic dissection 82, *82*
  endocarditis 77, *77*
  indications for *126*
  intra-atrial thrombus 49
  prosthetic valves 67, *68*, 70
  RV dilatation *93*
transposition of great arteries 102–5
  congenitally corrected 105
trauma, blunt or penetrating *121*
tricuspid annular plane systolic excursion (TAPSE) 91, *91*, *92*
tricuspid annuloplasty 72
tricuspid annulus 89
tricuspid regurgitation 59, 59–61, *60*, *61*
  PA systolic pressure estimation 94
  RV dilatation 90

tricuspid stenosis 59–61, *62*
tricuspid valve
  causes of disease *59*
  prostheses 72, *73*
  rheumatic disease 48, 59
two-dimensional (2D) echocardiography
  intracardiac dimensions *130, 131*
  measurement sites *129, 131*
  standard measurements 2
  standard views 1

urgent clinical advice, indications for *125*
urgent echocardiography 120–1

valve disease 39–64
  congenital 106
valves, heart
  descriptors in congenital disease *102*
  masses attached to 115, *115*
  prosthetic *see* prosthetic valves
  vegetations 75, *76*
velocity time integral (VTI1), subaortic *7*, 7–8
ventricles, assessment in congenital disease 102–5
ventricular septal defects (VSD) 100, *100, 101*
  post-closure studies *106*, 107
  RV systolic pressure estimation 96
ventricular tachycardia 122
views, minimum set 1–2

Wilkins score 49, *50*

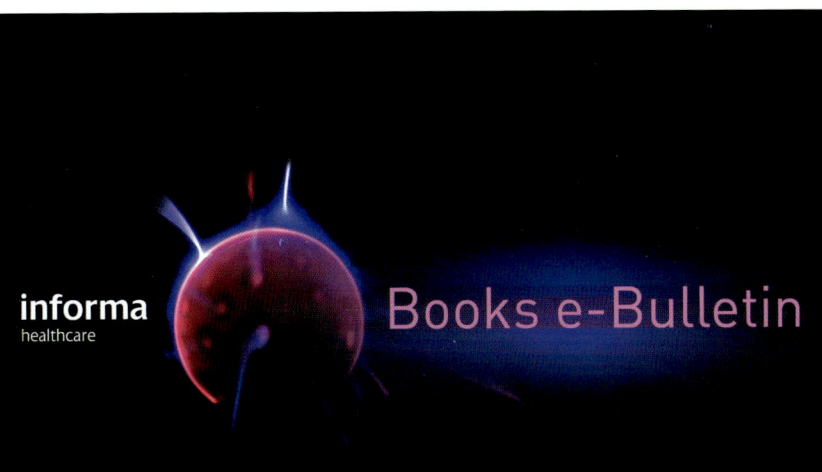

Key New Title from Informa Healthcare

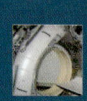
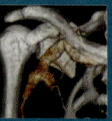

CT and MR Angiography of the Peripheral Circulation
Practical Approach with Clinical Protocols

Edited by **Debabrata Mukherjee** and **Sanjay Rajagopalan**
Respectively Gill Heart Institute, Division of Cardiovascular Medicine, University of Kentucky, Lexington; Mount Sinai School of Medicine, New York

Multislice CT has significantly increased the applications of clinical CT imaging but its beneficial impact has been most evident in vascular angiographic imaging. The excellent team of editors and contributors discuss the basic aspects of multislice CT angiography with chapters on technical principles, basic scan technique for peripheral vascular imaging with multislice CT, image reconstruction with multislice CT, radiation doses and contrast agent administration. Clinical applications for each major vascular territory are then discussed in depth, with clear descriptions of the examination technique for assessing the peripheral vasculature including the aorta to detect various vascular pathologies. A large number of high-quality illustrations help to explain the clinical findings making this text particularly attractive to the practicing clinician.

The section on MR angiography provides a comprehensive overview of the current state of magnetic resonance (MR) vascular imaging. The basic principles and technical features of MR angiography are outlined, with chapters on fundamentals of MR angiography and commonly used pulse sequences and contrast dosing. Specific chapters focus on each particular vascular territory including the extracranial and intracranial circulation, the pulmonary circulation, the thoracic and the abdominal aorta, the renal, and mesenteric circulation and both the lower and the upper extremity circulation. Easy to follow clinical protocols for angiographic imaging for the different vascular regions are provided. The text also addresses imaging of the venous circulation using MR and CT angiography.

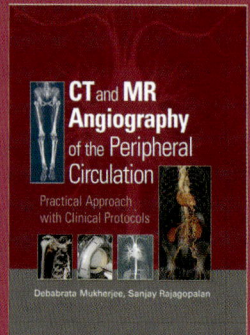

April 2007
H/b: 334 pages: 310 Illustrations
ISBN: 978-1-84184-606-4; **£145.00**

To receive regular email updates within your field subscribe to the monthly books eBulletin from Informa Healthcare. Visit www.informahealthcare.com/books/ebulletin to subscribe!

LIBRARY-LRC
TEXAS HEART INSTITUTE